The Effective
Weight Manager

FRED S. KUMMER

THE EFFECTIVE WEIGHT MANAGER

*A strategic weight-control system
and lifelong program
for health and success
with goals and objectives
that can be achieved
by every manager*

CONTINUUM · NEW YORK

1986
The Continuum Publishing Company
370 Lexington Avenue, New York, N.Y. 10017

Library of Congress Cataloging in Publication Data
Kummer, Fred.
    The effective weight manager.

    1. Reducing diets.   2. Executives—Psychology.
3. Executives—Nutrition.   I. Title.
RM222.2.K86   1986   613.2'5   85-29162
ISBN 0-8264-0365-4

To all who have desire and determination
to succeed in personal weight management:
You *can* be an effective weight manager.

Contents

Acknowledgments

Everyone at HBE Corporate Headquarters in St. Louis was excited about the writing of this book and I appreciate their enthusiastic support.

Particularly I want to thank the members of the Control Group Team: the people who tested the Strategic Weight Control System. Their questions and comments were invaluable to me and I must also single out for special mention the HBE corporate communications department for their efforts in compiling data and disseminating information.

Lastly, thanks to Dr. Arthur Zahalsky, biology professor at Southern Illinois University, Edwardsville, and Dr. Raymond R. Walsh of St. Louis University for their research direction.

Self-Management: The Bottom-Line Responsibility

"A manager must manage."
—from *Managing* by Harold Geneen

I don't think most people understand what they want from life or how they're going to get it.

Oh, they may have vague aspirations, such as: I want to be a successful manager. I want to be thinner. I want to be happy.

But the problem with their aspirations is those nebulous words: *successful, thinner, happy.* How can you define your goals unless you use precise terminology? How can you keep yourself on a path toward progress without an accurate system of measurement?

Managers who are good at their jobs, who do accomplish their goals, have developed clear definitions of what they want to accomplish. They are constantly tracking their progress by measuring in some reliable way the size of the steps they are taking. In short, they are constantly aware of where they stand in relation to where they want to be.

I have been described as "successful" by other people. They apply this label to me because I am the chief executive officer of HBE, a company I began in 1960 with

$18,000, which now has eight divisions, an annual payroll of approximately $27 million, sales in excess of $370 million a year. As owner of the Adam's Mark Hotels, HBE has become even more visible in the last decade.

It's very easy to measure success once a company or a person has become visible, once something has been demonstrably accomplished. In our society, dollar figures are the bottom-line measurement of success.

But long before anyone had ever heard of Fred Kummer or HBE or the Adam's Mark Hotels, I was a success—because I was managing my professional life, moving a step at a time toward the place I wanted the company to be. (And we certainly aren't there yet!) By applying the same principle to weight loss, I began successfully managing my weight before anyone noticed that my clothes were hanging loose, that my middle-age paunch was disappearing.

You *are* successful, thinner, happy—whatever you want to be—as soon as you make up your mind to be. When you decide, I know exactly what I want, then you move toward achieving it. To succeed, you need only two things: a genuine desire and determination; and some concrete means of measuring your progress toward your goals.

When I started my own firm in 1960, Kummer Construction Company, as it was known then, had one president and two employees, including my wife, June, an architect. We survived on nickel-and-dime jobs—a donut shop, a little church, a small neighborhood school. But I knew, in general at least, what I wanted to accomplish. I didn't want ours to be yet another small firm that turned out its yearly quota of small jobs.

It took six years to get the chance we needed to prove what we could do. An old college friend, an architect, came to me with a problem. He was designing a nursing home; and he couldn't manage to make the project cost-effective.

He said, "Fred, I know you can do this if anyone can."

That nursing home project provided me entry into the rapidly expanding health care industry—where HBE would develop a considerable reputation. The competition wasn't very effective at cutting costs. We were prudent in terms of our resources. I could cut 40 percent of steel tonnage out of a building, which amounts to 160 tons of steel, without lowering quality or safety standards—and nobody else could do that.

Kummer Construction began getting a lot of jobs. By 1973 we had so much work in this field, we changed our name to HBE, Hospital Building and Equipment Company. We could give clients the same building they could get from other firms at a fraction of the cost. We became the world's largest firm specializing in planning, designing, and building health care facilities.

And we did all that because we were—and still are—constantly aware of where we stand every day on every project we handle.

When I sit down with members of my staff in a meeting, I expect them to know exactly, right down to the pennies, where we are. The reason the construction industry—and most other industries, from movies through automobiles—frequently produce projects that come in over budget is a basic failure of accountability. The people who manage these projects somehow lose control of them, so they blame "uncontrollable" external forces for cost overruns. What has really happened is very simple: They have lost track of where they stand.

Our philosophy at HBE is: *You never lose track.*

Harold Geneen said it best: "A manager must manage." If a manager is not constantly on top of every aspect of his job, he isn't managing. He may be "working hard" or "keeping busy"—but he isn't managing.

Management requires constant awareness. There must

always be an exact accounting in every area of the manager's concern. If you adhere to this principle, nobody has to tell you how many hours a day you need to work or what you need to do to get ahead. You know what must be done, what has been done, and what remains to be done. At all times, you know where you stand.

People who successfully manage their personal lives always know how much money they have in the bank, how tall the grass or the pile of unwashed laundry is, how much they weigh. They manage through a system of personal accounting because they know if they don't, their checks will bounce, their lawns grow wild, their closets will empty, and they will gain too much weight to wear the clothes in those closets anyway.

Most of the books filled with management advice could be reduced to such simple terms. Yet authors attempt to tell readers what to wear to the office and how many hours to sit behind the desk, as if those were magic formulas for success. They aren't.

The formula is simple. You must control external forces, not let them control you—and determine your future. You must manage, if not master, your job and your life.

My critics—and believe me, all successful men do have critics—contend that HBE has grown to the size it has because Fred Kummer is a no-frills man, a pragmatist who delivers a basic product that is not innovative in design. To that last, I respond: Hospitals are not meant to be architectural monuments. They are meant to be cost-effective, to meet the needs of patients and staffs, not to please the aesthetic sensibilities of passersby. HBE has succeeded by always keeping these goals in mind, by never losing track of them, never allowing personal ego to interfere with the client's best interests.

As to the first part of the criticism: It's basically true. Fred Kummer is a no-frills man, a pragmatist.

It's easy to be seduced by frills and allow them to distract you from the basic management goal, in business and in life. And it's easy to kid yourself too. A lot of people work very hard for a little while. They keep their goals clearly in mind and move determinedly toward them. Then, either they have accomplished a little and begin to relax—or they have accomplished nothing and begin to despair. And they lose track of where they're at and they begin kidding themselves.

You know the syndrome: You turn in a quarterly report a little late and tell yourself it wasn't your fault because someone else didn't get you the material you needed on time. Or you gain a few pounds and tell yourself you really don't look so bad after all.

It's easy to kid yourself. Or let the frills take over your life.

Certainly "frills" have a place in one's life. I enjoy good wine, and I have a wine cellar of thirty-five hundred bottles. My wife and I are contemporary art aficionados; much of our collection is displayed in HBE world headquarters in Saint Louis, where we can share the pieces we love with the HBE family and clients who visit us.

But I would never let my pursuit of those interests, however pleasurable, distract me from business goals—or never let personal ego, mine or that of my staff, interfere with the accomplishment of a client's goals. At HBE, we value *management* ahead of everything else.

Of course we have grand illusions too. If we didn't, we would still be Kummer Construction Company, carrying out nickel-and-dime jobs. But we are very pragmatic about how our visions of the future will be achieved. We know you get to the end of the rainbow by taking little steps, one after another, by making the right decisions every day—not by making grand leaps of the imagination. We know those steps must be plotted and counted. Thus we always know how many steps we have taken and how many are yet ahead of us.

When we went into the hotel business in 1973, some people warned us that hotels are not like hospitals and can't be built in the same way. We know people go to hospitals and hotels for different reasons, expecting different services. But we also know the basic principle of management applies to both industries: daily accountability. We could have moved very quickly into the development of hotels and have far more than seven properties now—if we were willing to cut corners on that principle. But we didn't want to give up control. And that is what you have to do if you're going to grab every single opportunity down the road.

If management doesn't manage, if management doesn't control through keeping constant track of every detail—it doesn't manage at all.

A lot of hoteliers talk about how much they intend to do in the next few years. I am not concerned about the next few years. But I want to make sure that in twenty years the Adam's Mark will be an important hotel force in the country.

A lot of dieters talk about losing ten pounds in ten days or five pounds a week. When I started losing weight in November 1984, I wasn't concerned about the first five or ten pounds, the first one or two weeks. I knew I wanted to reduce from 188 to about 160 pounds.

If you know where you want to go, you can get there. The underlying principle is always the same: continuous accountability. It's the bottom-line responsibility of management.

Designing a Successful System

> " . . . the right answer (which usually cannot be
> found anyway) is not central. Central is under-
> standing of the problem."
> —from *Management* by Peter F. Drucker

I n the fall of 1984 I began to admit I was overweight.

Until then, I had convinced myself, as many people do, that I was "too busy" to watch my weight. My business demanded too much of my time for me to worry about the extra twenty pounds I'd gained over a ten-year period. Besides, I had grown accustomed to the comforting presence of a spare tire around my waist.

And I felt "fine." When I looked in the mirror, I looked "fine." Of course I didn't look in the mirror until I had knotted my tie and put on my suit coat. I was really kidding myself about how I felt and looked, what shape I was in.

I weighed 186 pounds. Since I am in my mid-fifties, and five foot nine, 186 pounds did not seem like an impossible amount of weight to carry around. Certainly I was not obese, not even fat. I was "just a few pounds" overweight, like the majority of Americans, including successful business people. I didn't think about weight beyond the brief nagging suspicion I felt whenever I stood in front of the mirror and reassured myself about how "fine" I looked.

Then one evening I was studying the quarterly reports on a profitable division of HBE. I noticed an area where we could cut some of the operational fat from the division and save several thousand dollars per quarter. I made a note to speak to the division head in the morning and continued reading. But the word *fat* stuck with me.

After my shower the next morning, I got on the scale. My weight was up a pound, to 187. Since I don't believe in worrying about weight fluctuations of one or two pounds in either direction, I didn't pay attention to this additional pound. Then, as I was shaving, I remembered the financial discovery of the night before. The word *fat* kept dancing around in my head. Like all great, and small, leaps of imaginative connection, this one happened instantly: *I was successfully managing a multimillion-dollar corporation by continuously monitoring the bottom line, but I was not managing my own body.* I had been ignoring the bottom line, the figures on my bathroom scale, for the past ten years.

Over the next few days I began to think about losing weight. I wondered if I couldn't apply the basic principle of management to weight control. After all, weight control is really nothing more than maintaining a state of constant awareness. People who successfully manage their weight are always aware of how much they weigh. The many choices they make each day about *what* they eat, *how much* they eat, and how they *expend energy* are determined by this underlying knowledge, this state of constant awareness.

When I thought about it this way, weight control seemed to be a process of monitoring numbers. The majority of us manage our finances successfully—because we are always, consciously or not, monitoring the numbers, the money in our checking and savings accounts, the credit line on our credit cards. We know if we can afford a $500 luxury purchase or not, if the budget will expand to include a second car payment or it won't. Personal financial monitoring is an inherent part of our lives.

We are aware of our professional standing in much the same way. Strong performance reviews, periodic promotions, fancier job titles, and larger office quarters are all measurable ways of telling us where we are in our careers. But salary, that all-important numerical measure, is probably the most significant way we have of monitoring career progress—and also of knowing where we stand in relation to others within our company or our field. What successful person isn't constantly aware of his or her measure on this yardstick?

Then why, I asked myself, can't we honestly monitor and control our weight in the same way we do our finances and our careers—when we have a basic and reliable means of doing so in our bathroom scale?

I began to see that I should manage my weight as I managed my corporation. And I wasn't. My weight at this point was up to 188. If a division of HBE operated with as much fat as I was operating on, I would never have ignored it the way I had ignored my waistline. I know the lean company is the profitable one. And I'd read enough about good health and nutrition to know the lean body operates profitably too—with less risk of disease and increased odds of a long and healthy life.

At that point, I knew I could develop a strategic weight-control system that was as basic as the bottom-line principle of business management: continuous accountability.

Analyzing the Competing Strategies

> "Fads and fashions in management theories, like
> fads and fashions in clothing, come in and quickly
> go out of style."
> —from *Managing* by Harold Geneen

First, I took a good look at the competing strategies, a representative sampling of the thirty thousand diets and weight-loss plans that are part of a $15 billion-a-year industry—an industry that thrives on fads and fashions.

The strategy common to all those programs is this: They are marketed as management miracles, radical changes in eating habits that promise long-term gains but in fact can only deliver *short-term* gains. All of them can work in the short run. Thus they do produce "miracles," but miracles that burn out faster than a thwarted takeover plan. None of them work in the long run.

I wouldn't spend twenty minutes with someone who promised me a business-management miracle, nor would you. We both know that no secret strategy, no instant management tool, will double productivity or triple profits in ten or twenty days. If someone told us we could take a small company and put it at the top of the Fortune 500 list in three weeks by developing a dramatic three-week growth plan, we would laugh, wouldn't we?

And most of us are equally suspicious of medical miracles—"cures" for diseases that have no real cures. Obesity is now regarded as a disease. Like alcoholism, it can't
really be cured. It can only be managed. Would a treat-
ment professional tell an alcoholic he could be cured by
participating in a short-term program? No. Yet "diet
counselors," a euphemism for diet salespeople, sell cures
every day.

The purveyors of diet pills and formulas and the authors of many diet books make millions of dollars on those
promised cures. They are selling the concept of instant
weight loss. People who would never buy the concept of
instant management lay their credit cards down for this
one because they *want* to believe. I understand why they
do. We have never been given a simple, workable system
for managing our weight. No wonder we are prey to the
sellers of short-term strategies.

When I began the research that led to the development
of the Strategic Weight-Control System, a sustainable plan,
I too examined the fads and fashions in dieting with some
degree of hope. I did not want to diet, yet I was prepared
to do so if I found a diet that didn't sacrifice long-term
goals for the short run. Immediately I rejected a batch
of diets and "weight-loss aids" on the grounds of common
sense. They ranged from out-and-out quackery—a "sauna"
suit, a $300 plastic ear form that is supposed to reduce
appetite when pressed—to diets that focused on one or
two foods to the exclusion of all else.

The Beverly Hills diet permits the dieter nothing but
specific fruits eaten at certain times of the day for the
first ten days. The F-plan diet, the rage of 1984, is a high-
fiber diet featuring fruits, vegetables, and grains. (Like
Dr. David Rubin's high-roughage reducing diet, which is
based on bran, it can lead to discomfort while sitting at
a desk, which most of us do.) The banana-milk diet requires bananas and three glasses of milk plus vitamin

supplements daily. Kempner's rice diet features only rice and fruit. Can you imagine ordering two bananas and a glass of milk at a business lunch? Or subsisting on fruit and rice while you prepare and serve delicious meals to your family?

Even if I could lose weight on such a regime, as undoubtedly I could, I considered twenty extra pounds preferable to a diet of rice and fruit.

The body-type diet divides everyone into four categories, based on where we store fat. It makes as much sense as dividing all the companies, large or small, into four basic types. According to this diet's author, each body type finds his caloric downfall in a different food group, for example, sweets, or starches, or salty snacks. Thus he devised a different eating program for the four groups.

I couldn't pick my body type from the illustrations of overweight people. I thought I might be a combination of two or perhaps three; and I didn't honestly believe I had accumulated twenty pounds because I overate in a certain "downfall" category. I had always eaten a balanced diet; I was simply eating too much of it.

I knew the group approach to weight loss, which involves behavior modification and weekly monitoring in a group setting, wasn't for me either. I am frequently out of town. And I am too independent, as I suspect you are too, for the group-therapy approach.

A friend who belongs to one of the weight-loss groups dreads Wednesdays, the day she must weigh in on the scale in front of her group. On Mondays and Tuesdays she starves herself and sometimes takes diuretics and laxatives in preparation for the weigh-in. On Thursdays and Fridays she overeats; by Saturday she is feeling guilty and beginning to dread Wednesday again. She reminds me of a manager who works frantically on two days each week trying to catch up with the work he didn't do on the two days he loafed. Obviously he will never catch up.

Next I looked at the supposedly "natural" or "health food" miracles. A few summers ago starch blockers were the miracle of the moment. They got more magazine play then MBO, management by objectives, if for a shorter time. These pills, composed of ground kidney beans, were supposed to block the body's digestion of carbohydrates. The manufacturers promised we could swallow starch blockers, eat all the bread and pasta we wanted, and *lose* weight. During the peak selling week of their short season, five million pills were sold.

You can't buy starch blockers now. Proven totally worthless by the Food and Drug Administration, they were removed from the market. But you can buy other miracles of the moment—Chinese teas; amino acid tablets, which advertisers promise will help you lose weight while you sleep; and spirulina, algae tablets that are supposed to kill hunger pangs.

Since I was familiar with the medical establishment's prohibitions against diet pills and liquid diet plans, such as the Cambridge diet, which dramatically restrict caloric intake, I rejected those strategies out of hand.

I began to read articles in popular magazines and medical journals about dieting, searching for strategies with more promise. The more I read, the more I disliked the word *diet*, which has negative connotations. I wanted a positive approach to problem solving, not a narrow and negative reaction to a condition, overweight, which most diet authors have apparently already decided we can't manage. None of the plans and programs helped people take control of their own weight. None showed respect for individual differences in management technique.

Could we take a generic five-year plan, apply it to all companies, and expect to thrive? Could we expect every manager within a company to respond in exactly the same way to a given problem? Of course not.

Yet dieters are led from one rigid "true plan" to another. When they fail to lose or they regain the weight they have lost, *they* have failed, not the plan.

Not surprisingly, some of these plans are almost mystical in their approach to weight loss, combining sacrifice and a near superstitious belief in the efficacy of eating certain foods at certain times of the day. For example, according to the developers of the Magic Mayo Grapefruit Diet (which is in no way connected with the esteemed Mayo Clinic), the eating of a half a grapefruit before each meal will magically "burn fat."

My own doctor, whom I consulted at the beginning of my weight-loss program (as anyone who plans to lose weight should do), assured me these claims were as false as logic told me they were. Moreover, the claims were in many cases dangerous. He put me in touch with authorities who shared their research on the results of fad diets. People who eliminate entire food groups from their diets or restrict their caloric intake below 1,000 to 1,200 calories a day for any extended period of time run the risk of developing serious health problems, including shock and low blood pressure, diarrhea, hair loss, high blood pressure, dehydration, abnormalities of the heart and nervous system, even sudden death.

Six such deaths and 138 documented cases of serious illness did occur among the six million users of the Cambridge diet plan during the spring and summer of 1984, the height of the diet fad's popularity.

I learned that even a doctor's name on the diet plan is no guarantee of its safety. Two diets developed by medical men have not withstood the rigors of performance review by the medical establishment. Dr. Stillman's quick inches-off diet (heavy carbohydrate, low protein) and Nathan Pritikin's maximum weight-loss diet (severely restricts calories and fats, also limits proteins).

Yet, in spite of the documented risks, VLC (very low

calorie) diets are popular. They promise to melt away fat and promote rapid weight loss. Very seductive promises. And most of us know someone who did lose weight by employing such a strategy. Of course we don't know anyone who has kept the weight off. But we are only too willing to blame the dieter, not the diet, aren't we?

Maybe, I told myself, a modified VLC would be worth the potential risks if pursued in short duration. I had examined the risk factors and was ready to view such a strategy as a high-risk investment, much like putting venture capital into a start-up operation. But I was looking for a potential investment with a good chance of success. If it could be compared to a tax shelter, I didn't want a shelter the IRS would disallow.

I began to gather research material that focused solely on the different diet plans' varying degrees of long-range effectiveness, not their medical soundness. I planned to consider the risk factor and inconvenience elements as the downside and balance them against the overall success ratios. The results were startling. The IRS would allow none of these as tax shelters, because the odds for long-range success are virtually nonexistent.

Put in another context, if these diet manufacturers were producing durable goods or selling services, they would all be out of business. They have the most dismal bottom-line percentages I've ever seen. And the results are made even more shocking by the nature of their business.

On any given day someone is trying to diet in 45 percent of all American households. Dieting is a national mania. Excess weight is a health hazard on a scale only recently acknowledged. In early 1984, a federal panel finally declared obesity a disease.

So how well is the $15 billion-a-year diet industry, which is an essential industry, succeeding in its objectives? *Of all who diet and lose this year, 95 percent to 99 percent (depending*

*on the study cited) will regain their weight loss within two years.
And five years later, one-third to one-half (again, depending on
the study cited) will have gained more than they lost.*

Deeply troubled by these statistics, I sat alone in my
office at HBE surrounded by the results of study after
study conducted on dieters who had attempted every con-
ceivable weight-loss plan. Why did they lose weight only
to regain those pounds and more? I thought about employees, friends, relatives, people who had worked hard
at losing ten, twenty, thirty pounds or more, only to have
those pounds creep back on as soon as the diets ended.
I had always wondered what was wrong with those people.
Now here was the evidence: There was nothing wrong
with the dieters.

Before I could develop my own system for weight management, I had to understand exactly why all these diets,
plans, and programs had failed. Obviously they don't fail
because they don't work. In fact, they do work. Follow
any one of them and you will lose. Yet none is based on
sound management practices.

They fail because they set up a pattern of failure. *They*
manage you for the short term. They don't teach you
how to manage yourself for life. Although short-term
gains are dramatic and satisfying, they are not sustainable.

Quick weight loss, those short-term profits, fool us
cruelly. The more quickly you lose weight, the more quickly
you will regain it. Much of the initial weight loss is water
and, unfortunately, lean muscle tissue—*not fat.* We lose
both fat and protein—but regained weight is mostly fat.
Cattle growers understand this principle: They under-
feed animals before fattening them to produce marbled
steak.

This lose-gain cycle, which is only profitable for cattle
growers, is called the yo-yo pattern.

You would not want to manage your business or your

checking account this way. Once you understand the pattern, you won't want to employ it in managing your body either.

The body responds to a diet the same way it would respond to starvation conditions: First, it conserves energy by lowering the calorie thermostat, the metabolism. And it jettisons water. The starving body reserves its fat cells as long as possible. Think of it as a badly managed company under siege from creditors. One by one the employees are "pink-slipped" to cut costs. Only the critical core staff remains. Your body regards its fat cells as part of that core.

As soon as you stop dieting and begin to eat normally again—*normally,* not even excessively—the body, which thinks it must now take advantage of the plenty in case starvation conditions suddenly develop again, regains weight on *less* food than before. Mounting medical evidence even indicates that this lose-gain pattern, not only the excess weight, is in part responsible for some of the diseases associated with obesity, mainly hypertension and diabetes. Not only do diets fail; they also may make us sick.

On-again, off-again dieters, those people who have "tried everything" and never achieved true weight control are simply the victims of their natural biology and a lot of bad management plans foisted on them by the quick-profit diet industry. They are not failures.

When I understood the yo-yo pattern, I was positive true weight control can only be achieved through a sustainable long-range plan, a plan that takes into account everything we know about the body's response to dieting. At this point in my analysis of the competing strategies, I read the book *Diets Don't Work!* by Bob Schwartz, a man who had reached the same conclusions about diets I had. I opened the book eagerly because I hoped he would have taken the conclusions one step further and developed a system. What he had constructed instead is a very complicated workbook, much like the workbooks of our school days.

His written exercises are designed to make us analyze our motives for eating. His is the *Psychology Today* approach to weight loss. People have undoubtedly lost weight working their way through his book—but what do they do when they finish the book? And what about all those overweight people, probably most of us, who will never have or take the time to complete essays on the specific conditions that led them to overeat?

Schwartz does have a program, rather than a diet; but the program is too complex. It does not provide the answers for the vast numbers of us who have gained weight through bad management, by simply losing track of where we stand. And finally, his program is not a system we can use for the rest of our lives.

My system would have to be based on long-term goals, on sustainable results. Although my personal use of the system would incorporate sound nutritional principles and a moderate exercise program, I was determined that anyone should be able to use it, lose weight, and keep it off even if he or she rejected good nutrition and refused to exercise. The people at HBE who volunteered to become the Control Group Team were going to test this requirement severely: They range in age from the twenties to sixty-plus, from five to eighty-five pounds overweight, from exercise addicts and health food nuts to those who will drive around the block for ten minutes waiting for a parking spot in front of the ice cream shop.

If the Strategic Weight-Control System could work for all of them, it could work for anyone.

The Control Group Team

"The significant difference between one manager and another is what standards each of them
sets, what each establishes to meet his own re-
quirements for satisfactory management."
—from *Managing* by Harold Geneen

A fter I began to lose weight, word spread around HBE
that Fred had a "system." One by one, other people who
wanted to lose weight approached me and asked, "How
are you doing it? What is your system? Will it work for
me?" Suddenly there was so much interest in the subject
of weight control among employees, family, and friends
I decided to write the system down on paper.

I wanted to share what I called the Strategic Weight-
Control System with as many people as possible, but before I did, I knew I needed to have it tested by a varied
group of individuals. Thus the Control Group Team was
developed.

I had mixed feelings about assembling this group. I
knew it was necessary to test the system on people who
had nothing in common but the desire to lose weight or
maintain a recent weight loss. I felt anyone could implement this system; and I wanted to prove this was true.

On the other hand, I believe so strongly in the concept of rugged individualism, which is basic to the system, that I did not want this "team" to think they were participating in a group that would attempt to manage their weight for them. I did not want them to see me as a weight-control guru who could help them manage their lives.

I also had to struggle with the conflict inherent in my role as the head of HBE. Would attempting to please the boss be a factor in their decision to test the plan? If so, they wouldn't be making a true commitment—and would they fail? It was important to me that no one felt obligated to lose weight, but anyone who wanted to learn about the system would have access to material.

I made every effort to dispel the notion that Fred Kummer would examine the questionnaires and know who was participating and who wasn't—that Fred Kummer would judge harshly the overweight person who had decided not to be part of this team.

Therefore, I had to keep a certain distance from the group. One of my communications managers took charge of coordinating the questionnaires and compiling the questions asked so that I could answer them, often with the help of medical authorities. She and I met frequently to discuss the kinds of questions the Control Group Team asked and the problems they had faced with weight control in the past, as well as the problems they still had. And frequently one of the group would stop me in the cafeteria or elsewhere to let me know how well he or she was doing or to make suggestions about items that should be covered in the material.

That was fine with me. I was always glad to talk about weight management. I wanted to be available to them; I just didn't want to force the system on anyone.

Many of the people who volunteered to test the system were the very people I would have expected to do so.

They had often complained about their weight problems when we were traveling together or they had commiserated with me when I would say, "I shouldn't have eaten that piece of pie. These pants are a little snug."

They were people who were overweight and knew it and felt unhappy enough to do something about it. In retrospect, we are all surprised that we weren't managing our weight as well as we were managing our jobs. Good management is so obviously the answer to weight control, we wonder now that none of us thought of it sooner. Why had we regarded overweight as a condition beyond our control for so long?

Pete, an architect in his late thirties, told me he gained twenty pounds every winter because he "couldn't help it." Yet somehow he lost those twenty pounds every spring so he could play amateur softball.

He said, "My diet approach is simple: I reach for iced tea, diet soda, or fruit when I want a snack. I stay away from carbohydrates and desserts. But as soon as I go off the diet at the end of softball season, I begin putting the weight back on again. Who can help gaining weight when the weather changes and the activity level drops?"

He laughed about his fluctuating twenty pounds, but he didn't really think his pot belly was amusing. I asked him if he would manage his job the way he was managing his weight—sporadically. For half the year, he responded to a crisis situation, the need to get in shape for softball, by managing. The rest of the year he didn't manage at all. If he handled his work in that fashion, not working some days, working overtime on others, what would his overall performance evaluation be?

When he put weight management in this context, he was appalled at his own management technique.

He wasn't alone. Other people had gained weight in response to changing situations in their personal or professional lives. Todd, a salesman in his late forties, gained weight when he got married. Paula, in her early fifties, gained thirty pounds after a medical condition forced her to withdraw from volleyball and bowling at the same time she switched to a job in food-preparation management. They did not recognize their bad management practices until they put weight control into management terms. As soon as they did, they knew they were allowing external forces or circumstances to manage them. They were reacting, not acting. They were *not* managing.

Some of them, especially those under forty, said they frequently put on ten pounds or so but were always able to take it off by stringent dieting. When they really wanted to control weight, they pulled out all the stops and did it. But were they managing? Or were they merely adept at accomplishing short-term goals?

A few of the Control Group Team were highly goal-motivated individuals who didn't look like they "needed" to lose weight.

Ron, whose weight was already in the "normal" range when he began using the system, wanted to lose ten or fifteen more pounds to increase his advantage in competitive tennis. Jenny, who appeared to be optimum size, wanted to lose the five to seven pounds she had gained gradually over a few years' time. Wisely, she realized she was *beginning* to lose control of her weight. And she wanted to take charge again before one day she found herself looking at twenty pounds of excess baggage, as I had done.

She wanted to find a lifetime system for maintaining a desirable weight. And so did Jeff, twenty-seven, who had lost 127 pounds several months before starting the plan. "I never want to be that fat again," he said. He also wanted to learn a technique of weight management that he could eventually teach his two small children. "I grew up with fat parents," he said. "And I became fat. I want my children to be in control of their weight, not controlled by fat."

Jack, at forty-eight, needed to lose weight for that very typical and practical midlife reason: high blood pressure. His doctor had ordered him to lose at least twenty pounds.

Most of the team had tried diets and exercise programs with varying degrees of success. Nearly all had lost weight and regained it. Joyce was typical of those who said their lives had been "a cycle of diets and periods of nondieting." She wanted to break the cycle forever. "I want a method of taking control at last," she said.

Carol, an ambitious manager in her early thirties, travels frequently, as do many of us at HBE. She wanted a system she could use on the road or at home. "Traveling is my downfall," she said. "I lose my good eating habits when I'm staying at hotels."

Each one of the group had the potential to become an Effective Weight Manager. I was convinced that they could and would achieve their weight-management goals if they had all the facts enabling them to make wise choices and a system that could easily be implemented in their lives.

I knew each one would have to accomplish this alone, for him or herself. The motivation for success had to be personal—the desire to look and feel as good as possible, to *know* that one is managing one's life effectively. I made it clear the Control Group Team was merely an assemblage of individuals, seventy-five separate Effective Weight Managers who agreed to share information on their progress if they could remain anonymous.

They were not a support group. And this was not to be regarded as another miracle cure, which would fail them over the long term.

5

The Irrefutable Data

"A problem well stated is a problem half solved."
—Charles F. Kettering

I n any business situation, a given, or set of givens, exists. You really can't analyze the options and make a good management decision without respecting the givens. In the business of constructing hotels, for example, the givens range from the very basic, such as the general purpose of a hotel (providing accommodations to travelers), to the specific factors of size and location, which vary from one project to the next. The givens determine the number of rooms, the cost of construction, and many, many other decisions. Often the givens are so obvious, we don't even think about them; but subconsciously we incorporate them into the planning process.

In the personal business of managing your finances, you also have certain givens. Annual income is the principle one. Who would think of developing a household budget that does not have this figure at its core?

The first thing a manager does, or should do, when confronted with a problem is examine the givens. He or she must decide what can be changed and what cannot. Very little cannot be changed by one means or another. Before anything can be done, the givens *must* be determined.

Yet we approach the business of weight management without knowing the givens, those basic facts that must be taken into consideration before we count calories, skip desserts, work out at the gym, or employ whatever means to lose pounds or maintain a weight loss. The set point, a relatively new concept, has become the bottom-line given of weight management.

Some of the Control Group Team members told me they couldn't lose weight because their set points were immutable. These people had decided their bodies were "comfortable" at weights that were more than they would like to carry. But, they insisted, they couldn't successfully fight their bodies' wills, could they?

They had taken the set-point theory on absolute blind faith. Some of us are naturally fatter than others, they argued; and there is nothing we can do to change it if our bodies "choose" to be fat. They were using the set-point theory the way too many managers use such reliable saws as "You can't teach an old dog new tricks." They used the set-point theory as an excuse for not managing their weight.

Yes, the set point is a given. It does exist in the same way your annual income figure exists. Of course you can't spend more than you earn without getting into financial trouble. And you can't eat more than your set point allows without gaining weight. But you can change the amount you earn if you are determined to do so; and you can change your body's set point too.

You can do this once you understand exactly what set point is, how it works, and how it can be regulated to your advantage.

A simple working definition of set point is: *the weight your body maintains naturally, without dieting.*

There *are* a few people who are "naturally" thin—no matter what they eat, no matter how little they exercise. Their bodies' thermostats are set to burn calories at a very high rate; and their metabolic rate (the function of this calorie-burning process) is likewise high. These people operate on a balanced energy budget that seems to require no management on their parts. But they may find themselves at midlife in the same position as most people because their set points may change. They may no longer be "naturally" thin.

Most of us are never so lucky at any point in our lives. We are not thin unless we manage our weight. And we are not content with the set points our bodies automatically regulate for us. We would like to regulate the system, if we only knew how.

And really we do know how: Balancing our energy budgets merely requires the same use of good management techniques we apply to the rest of our lives.

The set point determines the amount of fat the body will struggle to maintain in spite of your wishes. The cells that store fat release chemical signals to the brain. Those signals give little status reports on how much fat the cells contain and issue requisition orders for more fat. Glycerol, the chemical that helps bind fatty acids within the cells, is the messenger. Glycerol is a greedy messenger bent solely on requisitioning, not on balancing the budget, not on maintaining that all-important bottom line. The more fat in the cell, the more glycerol the cell releases into the bloodstream. The fatter you are, the more fat your cells request.

Think of those fat cells as department heads who have lost track of the supplies on hand. They keep requisitioning more. And the more supplies they get, the more they hoard.

Each body has decided it wants a characteristic quantity of fat and proceeds to balance food intake, metabolic efficiency, and physical activity to achieve that quantity of fat. The glycerol runs the errands. In response, the brain's computer will keep sending those supplies down unless a good manager writes a new program, cutting out the excesses.

That new program must respect the given, the set point, the irrefutable piece of data that does not go away simply because we try to lose weight.

Once you have established a low set point, a metabolic rate that is defending those fat stores, you are working with a particularly stubborn given. You cannot ever get rid of fat cells. They are not turned into muscle cells by exercise, as many people believe they are. Fat cells are not eliminated by calorie reduction either. Once you have added a fat cell, you have it for life.

Each fat cell can accumulate only so much fat. When all the body's fat cells are filled to capacity, the body doesn't simply stop adding fat cells. It forms new fat cells to accommodate the overload requisitioned by the glycerol messengers.

The poorly managed body continues to build new supply closets for supplies it doesn't need. The closets can never be eliminated. Fat cells can shrink, but they will never disappear.

So you are stuck with all those storage closets demanding supplies to fill them. It's tempting at this point to throw up your hands, yell "Set point!" and surrender weight management to the fat cells. When you consciously diet, refusing to supply the amount of food those cells want, the body responds by exerting less energy. It continues to protect the fat stores. You have written a new program, but the program doesn't work. No wonder you are discouraged.

Diets fight against the set point; and diets lose. The more severe the diet, the lower the metabolic rate drops as the body strives to protect its supplies. The irritability and depression you feel when dieting are the very real symptoms of the physical distress you feel at forcing your body to live below its set point. This is why dieters so often reach a plateau after a loss of ten or twenty pounds and seem unable to lose more, why they regain the weight they've lost when they stop dieting. Those empty closets are demanding to be replenished. Dieting doesn't change the master program, the set point, at all.

But the set point *can* be reset. The mindless management tyranny of the fat cells does not represent ultimate authority. *You* do.

A balanced budget, personal or corporate, takes into account the givens—which still leaves a wide range of choices. Two people earning the same amount of money each year will not choose to spend it in exactly the same way. Working with the same given, an annual income figure, they will develop vastly different budgets.

To balance the body's energy budget, you must acknowledge the given, the set point. From there, you have many choices. Activity level, food intake, and metabolic rate are the coefficients of set point.

If you are going to manage your weight successfully, you must manage fat storage. To do that, you must control the set point by balancing your energy budget. Focusing on the bottom line is the only way you have of measuring how well you're doing.

Most of us will find dieting alone a poor way of managing our weight. It probably will not have the desired impact on the bottom line. We will need to add exercise to change the set point. An active body is "set" to be thinner than an inactive one is. We'll examine the exercise options later and look at how the type and frequency of exercise affects the set point.

For now, we only need to understand that the set point does exist. But it doesn't have absolute power. Your body certainly can become "comfortable" with a smaller fat store. And you, not some chemical messenger, can be in charge.

6

The Discriminatory Policies

"It is doubtless impossible to approach any human
problem with a mind free from bias."
—Simone de Beauvoir

A savvy manager knows that discrimination, on some
level, will eventually be a reality in his or her professional
life.

"All things being equal" is a ubiquitous phrase that
seldom applies. All things are rarely equal, though we
would like to think they are. Managing a business, a career, or a family budget requires a pragmatic evaluation
of the inequities of one's circumstances.

The young MBA who isn't yet respected by his superiors, the older employee whose opinions are sometimes
discounted by youth, the woman or minority group member struggling to establish a career in a predominantly
white male field—all these people meet with prejudice,
however subtle or disguised. If they're wise, they will recognize prejudice and analyze what they must do to change
it or work around it.

They don't ignore prejudice simply because it should
not exist. A lot of should-nots do exist. Blindfold yourself
and you are apt to stumble on the should-nots.

You are probably not surprised to learn Effective Weight Managers have to deal with prejudice too. Unlike the corporate body, the human body has no antidiscriminatory policies regulating its behavior. In fact, some of the body's biological and genetic policies are widely discriminatory and totally impervious to logic. What I've discovered about the ways in which women and the middle aged of both sexes gain weight is unfair.

The average woman and the average man do not even store fat in the same places. Women tend to gain fat in the inner thighs and hips, men in the stomach, the region easily hidden by a suit jacket. New medical studies indicate that abdominal fat may have more serious consequences than fat stored in the hips and thighs. This may be in part why heart disease and arteriosclerosis are more prevalent in men than in women.

Obviously, fat is not an equal opportunity oppressor. Even the character of our fat may be gender related.

Fat deposits in males are sensitive to insulin, which causes men to gain weight more easily when under stress. Fat deposits in women are sensitive to the female hormones estrogen and progesterone (including the synthetic hormones found in birth control pills). And this is why pregnant or nursing women and those who take the pill put on weight. It also explains in part why menopause is also associated with weight-gain problems for women.

Helen, a Control Group Team member, who says she had "no problems" with her weight until she passed forty, calls herself "a victim of fat discrimination." She is afraid she can't be thin because she can't change "the fat facts" of her life.

"I retain water," she insists. "And I can't lose weight no matter how hard I try. My husband and I can go on a diet together; and he will lose weight twice as fast as I do."

Actually Helen isn't exaggerating.

Men can lose weight almost twice as fast as women do because they burn calories twice as fast for the same amount of exertion. With a higher proportion of muscle to fat, men burn fat more rapidly and efficiently. Muscle mass burns five more calories per pound simply maintaining itself than fat or connective tissue does. Fluid retention is also more common to the female physiology than the male.

So Helen is right: Women *are* born with the potential to be fatter, to be more resistant to weight loss than men.

Added to this obvious biological discrimination against her, Helen has a genetic disadvantage too. Her mother and father are both overweight. When both parents are fat, the odds are 80 percent that the child will be fat too. This particular genetic policy discriminates against men as well as women.

John, in his early fifties, insists he suffers as much, or nearly as much, from discriminatory policies as Helen does. He may be right too.

Both men and women past the age of forty require fewer calories to maintain their weight than they needed at thirty-nine, thirty-five, thirty. If they don't cut back on calorie consumption, perhaps by as much as 5 percent a year, or increase their physical activity, at least by a similar percentage, weight gain is almost inevitable.

"Middle-age spread" is no joke. It is real. We *are* programmed to gain weight as we age. And the discriminatory policies making us fat aren't restricted entirely to biology and genetics either.

John says, "I have a lot more career pressures now than I had when I was younger. I eat out of nervousness. And I have less time for regular exercise. And business meetings often include food. The facts of my life lock me into a weight-gain cycle. I really do feel out of control."

Helen counters, "Women are the chief preparers of food even in two-career households. It's hard not to taste when you cook. And increasingly working women are caught in the same time, exercise, eating-out bind as working men. Perhaps there really is no way around middle-age spread."

I told myself the same things when I was letting my body control itself. Before I became an Effective Weight Manager in charge of my weight, I found it easy to believe the irrefutable data, the set-point theory, and the discriminatory practices, which I vaguely recognized but hadn't clearly identified. And this made weight management impossible for me. I was behaving like the caretaker of someone else's company, not the manager of my own.

Like John and Helen, I was throwing up my hands and saying, "I can't do anything about it! Look at the givens! They're all negatives lined up against me."

Then I examined the discriminatory policies affecting me the same way I would examine a set of outdated regulations keeping me or my company down in some area— with an eye for loopholes. When I looked at them in this way, I was exhilarated, not discouraged. I admitted I couldn't manage my weight without respecting these facts. But I could also use them to my advantage.

I like a management challenge, as I suspect you do too. This is a *challenge*—not a barrier.

I believe I can solve any management problem as long as I am informed of all the facts, as long as I have all the options clearly in mind. At last I had the facts about weight. As a middle-aged man, I would have to overcome my body's prejudicial desire to be fat. I could; and I would.

7

Performance Review I

"... the number one motivator of people is feedback on results."
—from *The One-Minute Manager*
by Kenneth Blanchard and Spencer Johnson

The ubiquitous business meeting has several purposes other than filling space on executive calendars.

At the beginning of a construction project, for example, HBE people representing the various departments will meet to define objectives, develop time and cost budgets, determine whose expertise will be needed in which areas. As the construction progresses, our meetings will focus on problem solving.

A fairly typical business practice is to ask each participant to bring a written report to the meeting and share his or her work to date with the group. At this time, we at HBE often put unsolved problems before the group for discussion. We red-flag the trouble spots and make plans for dealing with them.

And, of course, business meetings also provide an opportunity for group members to reinforce each other's motivation.

The question-and-answer chapters located throughout

this book serve as business meetings between you, me, and the Control Group Team. Some of the questions asked by team members are unanswered. Their problems are shared. You will probably have many of the same questions and problems. I hope you can find the answers in these sections and also reinforce your motivation.

Q. Some diet authorities say we don't need a reliable means of measurement to lose weight. They say, "If you look good and feel good, if your clothes fit, you're okay." According to them, you can use these criteria to judge your weight. Why do you disagree with that?

A. For the same reason I would disagree with someone who told me, "We don't believe in accountants here at XYZ, Inc. We never know exactly where we're at. Our motto is, 'If we feel good, we must still be in business.' "

Without an accurate means of measurement, most of us will kid ourselves about where we stand. Remember, for several years I kidded myself that I "felt good" and "looked good" when I was twenty pounds overweight. It's just too easy to push those tight clothes to the back of the closet and forget about them. By the time you're buying new ones in a bigger size, you've lost track.

Q. But I do get diet conscious when I've gained five to ten pounds. Why isn't that level of awareness good enough? Why can't I just let things go until I am a little past my ideal weight, then diet? I've kept my weight more or less in line this way for years.

A. "More or less" is a totally unacceptable phrase to describe progress in a management situation, isn't it?

You aren't more or less on track, more or less within budget, more or less on deadline. Either you are or you aren't. Do you really think you're managing well if you don't begin managing until your weight is out of control?

How can you define an acceptable level of "out of control"?

Even in situations where you allow for a margin of error, you always know what that margin is. You always *measure*. I've never written or signed a contract in which specifications were preceded by the phrase "more or less."

Q. As long as I can drop ten or fifteen pounds on a crash diet whenever I want to do so, why do you say I'm *not* in control of my weight?

A. A crisis manager is only in control part of the time. The rest of the time he isn't managing at all. You may be able to "control" your weight now by crash dieting every time you gain ten or fifteen pounds, but in all likelihood you won't be able to do this forever. Eventually the lose-gain cycle will make you fatter. You will need to lose fifteen or twenty pounds, not ten or fifteen; and it will become increasingly hard to take that weight off.

Besides—and this can't be emphasized enough—you are jeopardizing good health by treating your body like a yo-yo. Would you run your business this way? No. You would never work hard to increase profits one quarter, then do nothing but spend the next quarter. Obviously the yo-yo approach to business management would bankrupt a company. What do you think it's doing to your body?

Q. I'm confused about what I should weigh. How do I determine my normal weight? I've compared tables published in magazines and newspapers and pamphlets in my doctor's office. The weights vary by as much as forty pounds in some height-and-frame groupings. What is right?

A. There is much disagreement in the medical community about the figures listed in the new tables. They do allow more pounds per inch than the previous tables did. It's tempting to accept the highest number you can find. But is that the weight at which you *really* function best?

Besides, these tables can be misleading. They do not necessarily reflect *ideal* weights but rather the average or mean weights of some specific group of people.

The 1983 Metropolitan Life Insurance Company height-weight tables (replacing the 1959 tables) are considered the industry standard. They were developed from data taken from the company's policyholders. Metropolitan issues this disclaimer: "The new tables do not necessarily indicate the weights that reduce the likelihood of illness, nor are they weights that optimize job performance or at which a person looks best. Because the weights are higher does not mean that people have a license to gain."

The tables are confusing. Perhaps the best way to determine your ideal weight is through consultation with your doctor.

Q. If we have trouble defining normal weight, how can we define obesity? Isn't it almost impossible?

A. I am surprised at how hard people—including myself at one point—will work to redefine "normal weight" and "obesity" to suit themselves. We would all rather be pleasingly plump than obese.

Obesity as medically diagnosed is viewed as anything more than 30 percent above normal weight—the weight your doctor, not a weight table, has determined is right for you. As you know, obesity is now regarded as a disease, so being honest about the definition has become a critical personal issue for all of us.

A medical researcher told me an amusing story about a former patient who was clearly obese yet objected to the diagnosis: "He insisted that, by his calculations using the new weight tables, he was only 28 percent overweight and not 30 percent. Thus he was not obese and his health was not really at risk. I told him he should consider using 'only 28 percent' as his epitaph so that people who walked past his tombstone would puzzle over its meaning for years."

Q. I'm finally ready to accept my situation: I am overweight. I have lost control, but I want to regain it. Fast. Why do all the experts caution against fast weight loss? Isn't fast better than slow?

A. You don't believe in get-rich-quick schemes, do you? Get-thin-quick schemes are nearly always as fraudulent.

The experts caution against fast weight loss for several reasons. Initial dramatic weight loss is largely accounted for by water and protein and lean muscle mass, exactly what you don't want or need to lose. Long-term weight management requires consistency; and no one can sustain a crash plan for long. In fact, starvation dieting boomerangs and makes you fatter.

You would not expect a business venture to pay off spectacularly for thirty or sixty days, then fizzle out. You would consider such a venture a bad investment. It's a poor way of managing money and a poor way of managing your body too.

Q. Why is there no one diet that works?

A. You are asking me why no utopian diet is capable of managing all of us.

We can't have a management model that works in every business situation we face. We have to make countless individual management decisions every day; and we make those decisions based on the data at hand, not on the sample data printed in a guidebook.

Diets don't work because they can't possibly compute that data. They try to make all the decisions for all of us all the time. And they try to make the same decision for the person who is ten pounds overweight and the one who is fifty pounds overweight, for the sedentary executive and the active mother of two toddlers, for the chocoholic and the guy whose downfall is pretzels and beer.

The model doesn't work. It can't work. Any rigid plan that does not allow room for independent decision making, for individual management, is bound to fail.

Q. But why are so many diets written by doctors or nutrition experts if diets don't work?

A. Sometimes the authors are well meaning; and the diets *are* effective at helping you take off weight, if not at helping you keep it off. Sometimes, too, get-thin-quick schemes do work—for the authors who can turn "thin" into "rich."

Q. I am too demoralized to try another diet. I have tried so many diets and weight-loss plans, including hypnotism, body wraps, cellulite creams, and pills. I have failed at all of them; and I hate myself.

A. Bad management *is* demoralizing.

When a company is badly managed, it's not profitably run. Everyone feels bad. People worry about job security. They feel helpless because no one is really running the company. It's out of control.

It sounds like you have bought too many weight-management theories. *They* have failed; you haven't. This time you are going to win.

Q. But I still don't understand why we can't find one secret, one management tool if you will, that makes weight management *easy*. Why can't it be effortless?

A. The "secret," if you insist on calling it that, is continuous accountability. This management tool requires us to be aware, to reason and thus control our weights. Perhaps that isn't totally "effortless."

But you wouldn't expect to be a good manager without exerting some effort would you?

We expect to work hard to achieve our goals in other areas. Why, in weight management, do we look for no-effort magic pills or potions?

Q. I have lost weight using diets before. And I don't know how I can lose weight this time without a diet. You say the Strategic Weight-Control System is not a diet. What about those of us who need diets?

A. If you want to use a "diet" within the system, you certainly may do so.

This time you will not be relying on the diet. You will manage the diet; it will not manage you. And when you stop "dieting," you will not stop managing.

Yes, you've lost weight in the past, but you've regained it, haven't you? And you regained it because you abdicated management responsibility to the diet plan for a period of time. When the diet stopped managing your weight, no one was in charge.

Q. I still don't understand why calorie counting fails. Shouldn't weight control be a very simple matter of counting calories?

A. Calorie counting fails because the calorie is not the accurate means of measurement it appears to be.

First, we do not always have the exact caloric measure of the foods we eat. For example, a bran muffin may be 150 calories or nearly 300. Unless you baked that muffin, exactly following a recipe that gives an accurate calorie count, you won't know.

When the calorie is our means of measurement, we tend to cheat. We "guess low" for foods. Even if we could *exactly* measure every calorie consumed every day—and we can't—we still couldn't accurately measure our bodies' use of those calories.

A calorie is "burned" when the body metabolizes it. Not everyone burns calories at the same rate. The rate at which calories are metabolized depends in part on fitness level, body fat level, and hormonal levels. Thus two people may eat the same amount of food but one will store more calories, the other will burn more.

An overweight person may have a low rate of dietary-induced thermogenesis (DIT), the rise in body temperature caused by the ingestion and digestion of food. The higher the body temperature, the more calories the body burns.

Calorie count is clearly not a reliable measure. Try to calculate profits from looking at a company's gross sales figures alone. Without knowing expenditures and that key bottom-line figure, the net, you are guessing at profits. Some guesses will be better than others. So it is with calorie counting.

Q. I've been trapped in the yo-yo cycle for years. Breaking the pattern seems impossible to me. I'm afraid I'm stuck. How do I get out?

A. If someone told you that you had to change a bad management practice or lose your job, you would change. We need to apply this same kind of mental discipline to weight control. We need to examine our real options and let go of weight-loss myths.

If we don't manage our weight successfully, we do lose the job. We lose it to external forces. I don't want to be managed by outside forces; and neither do you.

You can break out of the yo-yo pattern. First, admit to yourself that you are alternating periods of intense management (perhaps not self-management, but management by a diet) with periods of nonmanagement. You must practice continuous management now.

Q. I do a good job of managing my weight most of the time, but I lose control on weekends, holidays, when I travel or eat out. I don't see how that can change. I will have to carry those extra twenty pounds around with me. Besides, I associate eating with relaxing. If I am constantly alert, will I ever be able to relax?

A. I think you can relax without eating.

You are a situational manager; and you can change

that approach. Many authorities believe the most significant causes of overweight are behavioral: Those eating patterns we develop in childhood or that grow out of the routines of our adult lives. To say the behaviors can't be changed is like saying a company in financial trouble cannot be turned around by a good manager.

We know this isn't true. We've seen the dramatic results of turnarounds. Few of us are as pessimistic about the odds of improving lagging sales figures as we are about the odds for improving our own lagging figures!

Of course you can change—as soon as you take control!

Q. I was thin until I turned forty. I'm fat now. I can't get around the realities of aging and set point, can I?

A. You can "get around" those discriminatory policies as soon as you start working with, rather than against, your biochemistry.

Every one of us has had a difficult teacher or boss, friend or business associate. We learned how to please him or sometimes merely how to "get around" him. We couldn't achieve our goals working in our usual ways with this difficult person, so we found a new approach. As soon as you understand the discriminatory policies that in part govern weight, you will begin to find ways around them too.

Q. But I feel like a victim of my fat cells! If they'll never go away, how can I be thin?

A. They may never go away, but they can shrink down to the size of lean little storage closets you'll never notice. Managers are *not* victims. As soon as you start thinking like a manager, and not a victim, you will begin to wrest control of your weight from those fat cells.

Q. I have tried a lot of diets and lost a lot of weight on them, only to gain it back within several months of going off the diets. Why should your system be different? Why should I be able to keep the weight off this time?

The Strategic Weight-Control System will give you a tool, a very basic tool, for managing your own weight. All the diets failed because they never taught you how to manage your weight.

Suppose you hired a team of management consultants to run your company for a period of time because the company was faced with problems. That team worked from a secluded office; and they didn't share any of their management knowledge with you. You didn't know exactly what they were doing or why they were doing it.

When they left, the company was in great shape—for a while. Then, because you didn't learn anything about managing from those consultants, your company was in trouble again.

This time *you* are going to take charge of your weight. You will reach your goals and sustain that performance because you, not someone else, will become an Effective Weight Manager.

□ 8 □

Motivating the Team

"If you think you can win, you can win. Faith is
necessary to victory."
                                        —William Hazlitt

A companywide memo informed all HBE employees
about a brief meeting in the cafeteria after work. I emphasized that anyone interested in losing weight was in-
vited to attend and take home a packet of material, whether
they wanted to participate in the Control Group Team
or not. And I made it clear that we were not starting a
group-therapy weight-control program at HBE. This was
to be a plan for the individual, and I didn't want to present
it as anything else.

"The system is simple, but you have to use it exactly
as directed," I said. "You *can* lose weight if you apply the
same principle of bottom-line accountability to weight that
you routinely apply to work and personal finances."

I was especially concerned that they not believe their
success would be dependent on external support from
me, the group, or anyone or anything else, because it
isn't—no more than success in business management is
dependent on others.

I want you, the reader, to understand this too: *No one*

else can help you become an Effective Weight Manager; you can only do it for yourself.

This realization is absolutely basic to the program, a life-management plan that gives you the only tool you need for weight self-control.

Each one of the Control Group Team who volunteered to test the system did so knowing he or she was alone, not part of a support group. They had to develop their own independent equations for managing weight by balancing food intake and energy expenditure. The Strategic Weight-Control System would give them an accurate means of measurement. Other portions of the material we distributed would give them the information they needed to write those equations. They would have everything they needed to take control, but no one could take that control for them. Each one would have to make the decision to manage and stop *being* managed.

"The key," I told them, "is to rely on constant, accurate information about weight. You must stop kidding yourself about where you are. You must give up those nebulous terms and descriptions: 'I look fine,' 'I feel good enough.' You must define your weight-management goals and measure your progress as specifically as you define and measure economic goals."

They were perhaps confused about how to apply that advice, since they had not read the material you've already covered. But they saw how well the system was working for me; and they were excited about trying it. The best inspiration I could give them was opening my jacket and showing them the red suspenders holding up my once-snug pants.

As they filed out of the cafeteria and collected their packets of material, some stopped to chat. A few asked me how long I planned to "stay on the system." When I told them it was a system for life, they blanched.

"Does that mean depriving myself for the rest of my life?" one woman asked.

"No," I answered. "It means being in control of your weight for the rest of your life. I want to be an Effective Weight Manager forever. Don't you?"

She smiled and nodded. I'm sure she liked that concept of herself; and she should. An *Effective Weight Manager* sounds like a positive, active, take-charge person, whereas *dieter* conjures the image of someone who is deprived, denying herself the food she wants.

One problem with weight management in the past— for me, the Control Group Team, and probably for you— is simply that we never thought of weight in these positive management terms. Nobody expects to be a business manager for a few months, then quit. We *want* to be managers, in charge of our jobs, our finances, our lives. The word *manager* is not frightening to us. It's a strong term. Naturally we like the way it sounds.

Before you put the system to work in your life, I want you to think of yourself in this positive way too: You are a manager, not a dieter. You are becoming an Effective Weight Manager for life. You really are ready to take that step now.

Up to this point, we have analyzed the competing strategies, examined the irrefutable data of set point, and studied the discriminatory policies that affect the way each one of us will have to implement his own Effective Weight Manager plan. We have looked at the weight problems the Control Group Team has had in the past and identified the ineffective management styles they used. Probably you have recognized your own problems, named your own ineffective approaches to management.

We have discovered that diets fail because they attempt to manage us and don't teach us how to manage ourselves.

Through this analytical process, we have taken the myth

and magic out of weight management. As long as we believed weight control was dependent on external forces— whether those forces are a set point or a grapefruit diet that melts fat—we weren't managing our weight. Why should we? We had built-in excuses for not managing, fall-back positions for failure. Once we accept that weight control is self-control, management in its purest form, we *are* in control.

You have achieved that realization now; and you are on your way to becoming the size you want to be, to becoming an Effective Weight Manager.

What is an Effective Weight Manager's basic management function?

If someone were to ask you what is the first function of business management, you probably wouldn't have to think long before answering, "Economic performance." No matter what your role in a company, you always have, as the first objective, economic performance. If that goal isn't met, no second or third agenda exists. No one has a job.

That is the bottom line of management. Every decision, every act, has an impact on the bottom line—economic performance.

The first function of weight management is also performance—achieving and maintaining a weight that is healthy and desirable for you. Just as the success of a business manager can be measured in economic terms, the success of a weight manager can be measured in specific numerical terms: pounds.

As you become an Effective Weight Manager, keep in mind the integrated nature of management. The tasks of management—planning, problem solving, decision making—are interconnected, focused on results. A good manager is always aware of how the tasks connect and intertwine, of where he or she stands in relation to goals.

Now you will begin to apply that same level of awareness to all the decisions about food intake and energy
expenditure that affect the bottom line, your weight.

Admit it: For people like you and me, the worst aspect
of being twenty (or however many) pounds overweight
is the nagging feeling that one is no longer in control.
One of the last people to file out of the HBE cafeteria
after our meeting told me, "If I could just get my weight
under control, I would feel a lot better about myself."
Haven't you had the same thought?

The Strategic Weight-Control System

> "The greatest discovery of my generation is that
> human beings can alter their lives by altering
> their attitudes of mind."
> —William James

The Strategic Weight-Control System works because it
is not a diet.

I am not going to tell you to count calories, because I
don't count calories. I have neither the time nor the opportunity to follow a rigid eating regimen. And I assume
that you don't either. Busy people, especially those who
travel frequently and combine business with lunch or dinner, cannot successfully commit to a diet program that
requires them to eat a piece of fruit at ten each morning
or lunch on hard-boiled eggs and lettuce. Unless we can
check ourselves into a health spa or a fat farm for a month
or six weeks, we will have to continue ordering from
menus and making many conscious food choices each
day.

Business managers are used to making decisions every
day. Those decisions, large and small, determine how
they will divide their hours and expend their energies.
If they permit external forces to control their working

days, they are not managing. They are being managed. On the other hand, it's simplistic to assume that other people and external forces will never cause one to stray from the course originally set for the day. Sometimes we must change our plans—in response to a crisis or a better idea.

Managing your weight, then, is no different than managing your job. You have to make a lot of little decisions about what kind of food *and* how much of it goes into your mouth and whether you will walk up a flight of stairs or take an elevator. Sometimes you will give in to impulse or circumstance. You will eat a dessert or you will grab a take-out meal on the way home because you don't have time to cook. If you are rigidly following a diet, those little decisions will make you feel you have failed. You will decide you can't manage your weight after all.

But put your weight in management terms, and you will begin to handle it exactly as you do your job, checking account, investments. You will know what you have to do to reach your goal weight—by being constantly aware of where you stand. Through a system of continuous accountability, you will focus on the bottom line, not the dish of ice cream, the slice of pizza.

Weight control is a function of the three variables: what you eat, how much you eat, and how much energy you expend. *You* determine the percentage of each variable in your own weight-control equation. Some of us will choose to exercise more vigorously or more often than others. However you determine the equation, you do so without the guilt that is attached to diets and/or rigid exercise plans. You are always focusing on the bottom line, on *progress,* not on each individual choice you make during the day.

A good manager maintains control over the business as a whole. He doesn't know *approximately* the figures for payroll, sales, unearned income; he knows *exactly*. In the past, we haven't had that kind of measurement for weight control. We have focused too much on whether or not we "can" have a slice of bread, a pat of butter—and not on the bottom line, the numbers on the scale.

Most of us weigh ourselves once a week or more often, maybe even daily—as long as we like what the scales are telling us. I know a lot of people who say, "I weigh myself now and then; and that's how I control my weight." Or, "I know it's time to go on a diet when my waistbands are tight."

By the time your waistbands are tight, too much time has already elapsed. You have gained beyond your desirable weight. And you have begun kidding yourself about how you look. Maybe you put the tighter clothes to the back of the closet. You've stopped wearing a vest, those gray trousers, that sleek knit dress with the wide belt. And you've stopped weighing yourself because you don't want to face the numbers.

At this point, you have stopped managing your weight.

Maybe you are only five or ten pounds above an ideal weight. And maybe you're right when you tell yourself, "This isn't so bad." At least you may not look "so bad" to other people, who see you wearing the fuller clothes cut to hide the weight.

But you know the truth: You have lost control of your weight.

Well, I believe you are an intelligent person. If you have the information you need to make intelligent decisions, you will make them. And that is the heart of the Strategic Weight-Control System: Provide yourself with the information you need *every* day to make the decisions you must make about food, and you will make good decisions. You will manage your weight.

In the past, you haven't managed weight effectively

because you haven't measured weight with enough precision. Starting right now, you will work with a system of accurate measurement. Like a good manager, you will keep a good set of books.

Here's how the system works:

- Each day, at the same time every day, weigh yourself. I weigh myself first thing in the morning, as I think most people do. But the time of day you choose to get on the scales isn't important; only the consistency matters.
- Record this weight in a notebook each day.
- At the end of the week, average the daily figures. If you have not weighed yourself for a day or two, average the daily weights you do have by adding them, then dividing by the number of days you weighed yourself.
- Record this figure also.

And this is all you have to do, now or ever, to manage your weight.

The object is to keep the weight curve moving downward until the desired weight goal is reached. When this happens, you don't throw away the notebook—or the program. Just as a manager doesn't stop keeping track of business when sales are booming, you don't stop keeping track of weight once you weigh what you want.

Rather, the object becomes maintaining weight. You want to keep the weight curve more or less straight across the chart—for the rest of your life.

Carrying the notebook with you *may* help you, at least in the beginning, to maintain that awareness. I usually have mine in my suit pocket; and I find it does serve as a reminder of my long-term goals. But it certainly *will* help you to plot the weight line on graph paper. Watching the line curve downward will reinforce your determination—and it's fun, like winning a game. Also, unless you do chart the line, giving yourself visual support, you may find it difficult to think of weight management in terms of a graph line, which is the cornerstone of the Strategic Weight-Control System. At the back of this book is the graph I plotted over the twelve-week period in which I lost 11.07 pounds.

I don't worry if I wake up one morning and discover I weigh one pound more than I weighed the day before. That's going to happen. Maybe I've been out of town on a business trip. Maybe I went to a restaurant with my wife and some friends and I couldn't resist dessert. That's okay. I won't let this one day, this one restaurant meal, this one pound, convince me that my program is a washout—that I can't manage my weight. I *can*.

The slope of the line is what counts, not the occasional, brief upward fluctuation.

Each week while I was losing, my average weight was less than the average of the week before. Although I had an overall goal in mind of losing two ounces a day, I wasn't worried about those ounces every day when I got on the scale.

As long as I know exactly where I am every day, I am in control of my weight. My little notebook is like a bankbook. I compare my system to an accounting system. Yes, it is an accountant's or an engineer's approach to weight management: a system of precise measurement that does not inhibit your ability to respond creatively to the forces around you.

But because I know where I stand, I make better conscious choices about my meals. Maybe I will decide to skip bread or make my dessert choice fruit. It does not matter which individual choice I make. All that matters is the constant accountability, the daily information that allows me to keep the slope of the line going in the right direction. Diets fail because they try to anticipate all the choices—and make them for us.

I can hire a manager and tell him what his responsibilities are in his department, but I can't sit down with him every day, watch him every hour, and tell him what he needs to do to meet those responsibilities. If he is a good manager, he will make the right decisions.

This weight-management system accords you the same respect I accord the managers I hire. It assumes you are competent enough to make good decisions as long as you have accurate data. Without eliminating any foods from your diet, cutting calories in a conscious way, restricting yourself to set menus, you will reduce food intake yourself. You will lose weight simply through constant awareness of where you stand.

Once you know exactly where you stand at all times, you cannot fail.

□ 10 □

The Underlying Principle

"Eat regular, well-balanced meals with enough
variety to assure good nutrition."
— Jane Brody, *New York Times*
"Personal Health" columnist

Yes, you can manage your weight using the Strategic
Weight-Control System even if you choose to exist on a
diet of junk food. I promised you: No diets! But what
you may not manage so well over the long term on a junk-
food menu is your health. Good nutrition is basic to good
health.

Increasingly, we are learning how much nutrition contributes to health. We do need a selection of foods from
the basic four food groups: meat and fish, milk and dairy
products, fruits and vegetables, and grains. And according to some new research, we may even be able to prevent
cancer or heart disease by eating a low-fat, high-fiber diet.

Nutritional fads are being replaced by the balanced
diet, in vogue once again. Several years ago people believed a high-protein diet kept them healthy and slim, so
they ate lean meat, eggs, and cheese, and skimped on
carbohydrates, such as potatoes and pasta. Now pasta is
promoted as a health food. Although we need protein

each day, we also need carbohydrates. Protein, the only nutritional requirement the body can't meet in stored fat, keeps blood sugar even and satisfies hunger. Carbohydrates, natural sugars and starches, are a tremendous source of energy.

Once I became constantly aware of my weight, I also became highly aware of the kinds and amounts of food I put into my mouth. I had always heard some foods were "fattening" and others were not. Some were "good" for me; others were "bad." But what was the truth behind those words?

When I realized I could no longer afford to eat an excessive amount of food, I knew I needed to be aware of which foods were nutrient-dense and which were not, which were calorie-laden and which were not. If I chose a "fattening" food, I wanted to know exactly what I was choosing and how it was or was not meeting my body's needs—so I could balance that choice later. Of course no one is going to eat a perfectly balanced meal every time, but I wanted my meals for the most part to be well balanced.

I knew what a balanced budget was, but I was less clear about the definition of a balanced diet.

I talked with several nutritionists and learned most of us are not as well informed about food as we are about money or cars. The average person knows more about Independent Retirement Accounts and money market funds, about the depreciation value of cars and finding the best interest rate, than he does about the calcium content of broccoli or the protein value of cottage cheese. And a lot of what we think we know is misinformation.

For instance, no food is absolutely "fattening," and conversely, almost any food, eaten in sufficient quantity, can make us fat. We get fat from eating too much, exercising too little. Some of us get fat on balanced meals, others on Hostess Twinkies. We can't blame the Twinkies or the steak and salad.

Some of our cultural food myths include:

- Potatoes are high in calories.
- Margarine is lower in calories than butter.
- Yogurt laden with sweetened fruit is "diet" food.
- Washing spaghetti before cooking will remove calories.

None of these "facts" is true!

Yet the nutritionists tell me our fondness for misinformation is not as damaging as our taste for fat. Americans now eat 43 percent, almost half, of their calories in fat—well above the recommended daily fat intake of below 30 percent of total calories.

That traditional American diet (heavy on meat and potatoes loaded with butter, gravy, sour cream, or fried in oil) isn't the healthiest diet; and a growing number of us are making changes in it. Nutritionists advise: Cut back on red meat; eat more chicken and fish, preferably broiled, baked, or grilled; cut down on fried foods; add more fiber in the form of fruits, vegetables, and grains to the diet. In other words, many of the food choices we make every day in restaurants and fast-food outlets, employee cafeterias, and our own kitchens may not be "wrong," or "bad," or "fattening" choices, but the cumulative effect of making those same choices over and over again could be wrong or bad in nutritional terms—and certainly could make us fat.

It is possible to be overweight and malnourished at the same time. Can you think of a worse example of managing than that?

Nutritionists recommend that people on weight-loss plans take a multivitamin and mineral supplement each day to be sure they are getting necessary nutrients. They do mean *one* pill, not several. Vitamin megadosing is popular among some health food faddists, athletes, and others. Now we know that people who overdose on vitamins may actually be harming body organs and certainly aren't helping themselves. We only need a certain percentage of each vitamin or mineral per day. Unless your doctor has determined that you need more than this percentage, you shouldn't be taking it.

Since I had always taken one vitamin supplement each day, I merely continued the practice. People who eat little or no red meat or who exercise heavily and frequently (especially women) should take a supplement that includes iron. And some of us, especially women again, may need calcium supplements. Thin and small-framed women are particularly susceptible to osteoporosis, a degenerative bone disease that strikes postmenopausal women.

Aside from these supplements, no other nutrient pills are necessary unless prescribed by a physician. Those pills found in health food stores that contain seaweed or garlic oil and parsley, for instance, contribute nothing of value. They only waste money.

The more I learned about nutrition from experts, the more I realized that good nutrition is in large part good common sense. Limit consumption of caffeine, alcohol, fats, sugar, and salt. Eat three balanced meals a day, beginning with breakfast.

Have you ever wondered why everyone from your mother to diet authorities tells you *not* to skip breakfast?

The digestion of food starts a protein action that insures the chemical balance necessary in your body for burning fat. Overnight the whole process virtually shuts down. If you skip breakfast, your body won't start working again burning fat as efficiently as it would if you ate breakfast. And this only compounds the problems of late-day hunger for breakfast skippers. When you skip breakfast, you are often ravenous by lunchtime. You overeat. And your sluggish system isn't burning fat.

Another one of the nutrition axioms you probably heard from your mother may not be true: Don't snack between meals.

Snacking per se isn't "bad." If you save part of lunch and consume it as an afternoon snack, you aren't adding more food to the day's total. If you snack on potato chips, in addition to lunch and dinner, you are adding food—in the form of empty calories.

Most of us already know, however, that a bag of potato chips isn't good nutrition. We may not be aware of the exact calorie count of the chips, but we know they provide more calories and less nutrition than an apple does. But sometimes we are going to eat them anyway.

When we look at our food choices in this commonsense way, we can treat them like the management decisions they are. Food is not a reward. Nor is it a forbidden sin. It is an *expenditure*.

Every day you decide how to spend money. Some expenditures are not strictly necessities. As long as your basic living expenses are met, you are free to decide if your expendable dollars will go toward books or movie tickets, fishing rods or shoes. You can choose to take a long vacation or several short weekends.

We don't put those kinds of personal decisions into the same category as our food decisions. We should. We know spending money is a management decision; and most of the time, we don't assign a moral value to this type of decision.

We do assign moral values to food, and sometimes the moral values have little to do with nutrition. Donuts are "bad," but so we used to think is spaghetti. Celery sticks are "good." So is diet soda. We are virtuous if we make "good" choices; we are not virtuous if we make "bad" choices.

Those labels represent a kind of thinking that focuses on calories and obscures nutritional logic. That thinking turns food into something other than what it really is and makes food choices fraught with moral, rather than nutritional, meaning.

Food choices should simply be weight-management decisions. Again, once you are holding yourself continuously accountable for your weight, you will begin to make better choices. Only a few weeks after we distributed the Strategic Weight-Control System information at HBE, the cafeteria manager told me about some dramatic changes in the employees' eating habits.

Salad sales were up. Fried foods, especially french fries and onion rings, a favorite, were down. People were buying more baked fish, less fried. Overall, cafeteria sales were down $100 a day.

These people weren't conforming to a "diet." They were simply making better choices. So will you.

11

Performance Review II

" . . . eliminate the behavior and keep the person."
—from *The One-Minute Manager*
by Kenneth Blanchard and Spencer Johnson

Q. I've been weighing myself daily for years. I'm still overweight. But I know people who go to Weight Watchers, where they only have a weekly weigh-in; and those people are losing. Why?

A. Have you honestly been weighing yourself daily? Or have you perhaps weighed yourself *frequently?* Maybe you avoided the scale on the days when you were afraid the news would be particularly bad.

I weighed myself *most* days, too, before I developed the Strategic Weight-Control System, but those sporadic measurements were not meaningful to me on their own. Numbers are only meaningful in relationship to each other.

Many people who insist they weigh themselves "daily," upon more careful consideration, admit they do skip a lot of days. Weighing yourself on an occasional or even a regular weekly basis allows you too much room to manipulate the results. You can't gain an understanding of what the numbers mean in terms of your body. When you weigh yourself daily, record, average, and chart the weights, you see the tangible effects of a heavy late dinner or of skipping a workout, of consuming salt, sugar, or fat. You get to know yourself and how you are affected by every food and energy-expenditure choice made.

Possibly you have weighed yourself on a daily basis before you started using the system—but you were simply not paying enough attention to those numbers to assimilate the information they give you. The Strategic Weight-Control System forces you to look at the numbers in a totally new way. Numbers are the guts of a business. You cannot manage well without keeping constant track of them.

Q. I have always weighed myself when my clothes began getting tight. Then when I see on the scale how much I weigh, I cut back. I also try to cut back the day following a splurge like an ice cream sundae. Still, I am ten pounds overweight now. Why hasn't continuous accountability worked for me?

A. You haven't been practicing continuous accountability.

When you wait to weigh yourself until your clothes are tight, you've waited too long. You've lost track of where you are. Do you balance your checkbook each time you write a check, or do you wait until you suspect you've spent all the money in your account, then balance it to see how far overdrawn you are?

If you were in a retail business where you bought an item for five cents and sold it for six cents, you might think that if you had enough money to keep the doors open, you were profitable. The truth is you wouldn't know *how* profitable until you had calculated overhead and measured its impact on that one-cent margin.

If you don't weigh yourself until your clothes get tight, you only know you're still making some kind of profit—

that is, your clothes still do fit. You don't know what kind of profit you're making. You don't know where you stand.

Q. I was expecting a far more structured program. You say the advantage of the system is that I don't have to go on a diet, but I think I need more direction. I would like to have low-calorie meal suggestions and other aids. Why don't you give them?

A. You can find low-calorie meal suggestions in almost any women's magazine on the newsstands. They are dietician-tested and feature foods in season. I am not in competition with the women's magazines because they can do this particular job better than I can.

I am simply telling you that you will never lose weight and maintain that weight loss for life until you begin to *manage* your weight. I cannot manage for you by providing a highly structured program that will keep you in control for a short period of time. As soon as the program was over, you would be in the same place you are now: You would be nonmanaging.

Q. I have seen diet plans that tell you to keep food diaries in which you write down everything you eat every day. This is supposed to help one lose weight. What do you think?

A. I don't have time to write down everything I eat all day long any more than I have time to record every single out-of-pocket expense beginning with the morning paper. Do you? If you do have the time and want to keep a diary, you can. However, it is not integral to the simple Strategic Weight-Control System.

Q. Basically, isn't your message simply to cut down?

A. No. What do you mean by "cut down"? Can you measure and define that term? "Cut down" is another one of those nebulous phrases. I may tell you to cut down. So you may switch from eating three cream puffs at your coffee break to two—and still not lose weight, though you have "cut down." A specific system of measurement is necessary to a good management program.

Q. I have heard of programs where you chart your goals and enter your weight next to the goals to help maintain discipline. How is your system different?

A. The chart is only part of my system. Keeping the notebook is the critical element in the Strategic Weight-Control System's success. In the beginning, the chart will perhaps be more important to you because initial weight loss is usually greater and looks more dramatic on a graph. The line sloping down the chart will make you feel good about yourself, as it should.

Once you get deeper into the program and weight loss comes in smaller increments, the notebook will become more important to you. When I reached the point where I was losing a quarter pound or less a week, the chart didn't illustrate loss as dramatically for me as it once had. But the numbers in the notebook, as they fluctuated from day to day, told me a lot about myself. I achieved a self-awareness through that notebook in ways you will only begin to appreciate when you get there too.

Q. I don't see how I can possibly get a balanced diet and control my weight without consuming too many calories—unless I have information available about the calorie count and nutritional content of basic foods. Why don't you provide this?

A. Once again, the competition does it better. Have you seen those pocket calorie guides in the check-out lanes of the supermarket? If you want one, buy it there.

You can have an approximate idea of the number of calories you're consuming each day and an approximate idea of the nutrient contents of the foods you eat. You can't be exact about calories unless you are preparing every meal from scratch at home. You can't even be exact about nutrient content if you're doing that because nutrients in fresh foods, such as vegetables, are in a sense perishable. If a head of lettuce has been in the grocer's case for several days, it no longer has the same vitamin and mineral content as a fresh head.

By taking a vitamin supplement and eating from a variety of foods, you are assuring as good a nutrient balance as possible.

Again, the only exact measure we have available for weight control is the bathroom scale. The more you travel or dine out, the more this becomes true. Would you tell me you couldn't manage your job without an exact list of duties to be performed each day—accompanied by a sheet assigning time values to them? What you've said about weight management is tantamount to making this statement.

Q. I was shocked to read that my favorite triple burger at Wendy's has over a thousand calories. Don't we need this kind of information if we're going to lose weight? Why does your plan provide no information on fast foods? Aren't you ignoring them?

A. The Strategic Weight-Control System ignores nothing! I may not know the exact calorie count of a pizza, but I know what kind of impact it has on my weight. If I ate a small pizza every Tuesday night and every Wednesday morning my weight went up by one pound, I would know the most important fact I needed to know about that pizza.

Before you read the calorie count of your favorite burger, didn't you suspect it was more caloric than a single burger? Most of us have heard enough about the calorie content of fast foods to know we aren't getting calorie bargains when we line up for them. We are still free to make that choice using the system.

If I wrote a rigid diet program prohibiting you from ever again eating a Wendy's triple burger, would you follow it? Or would you still eat the occasional triple and feel guilty about it?

With the system, a triple burger is only one factor among many. *You* measure the total effect of all your choices daily. *You* begin to understand how each choice affects the bottom line. *You* manage.

Q. A lot of doctors say you don't need to weigh yourself every day on a diet. In fact, many say you shouldn't weigh daily because you get discouraged. I know I am discouraged. I weighed myself every day for a week and I didn't lose anything. I would rather stop weighing myself until I feel like I've taken off some pounds. I can't stand the bad news.

A. I disagree with the doctors who say you don't need to weigh yourself daily, because weighing daily works so well for me and others. You are discouraged because the needle on your scale hasn't moved and you want to avoid the bad news. Will you change the truth by ignoring it? Can you make a fact go away by not looking at it?

Managers are often tempted to take into consideration only the good facts, the ones they want to hear, the facts that will back up the decisions they want to make. But management requires fearlessness. You must face all the information, the pleasant and the unpleasant, and deal with it.

You must keep weighing yourself daily, recording and charting the weight. This is the only way you will keep track of where you are. Only through constant awareness will you begin to make the right management choices, which will enable you to lose weight.

How can you make decisions within the context of the bottom line if you don't know what the bottom line is?

I know daily weighing can be discouraging. No one can make progress every day. There were times when I had gained weight, times when the needle on the scale stayed in the same place for longer than I thought it should. Every manager knows this kind of frustration. And those are the most important times to practice good management.

Q. But I get bored with weighing myself daily. It seems like a chore. Isn't every third day good enough?

A. How long does it take to weigh yourself and record that figure daily? To average and chart weekly? Can you really get bored in such a short time?

Possibly you are fighting the concept of self-management, resisting the idea of taking charge of weight management completely. Try using the Strategic Weight-Control System, exactly as outlined, for three months—weighing yourself daily, recording the weight, averaging the figures weekly, and charting them. By the end of three months, you will become fascinated with what those numbers tell you about yourself, about the choices you are making, about what kind of impact those choices have on your bottom line.

12

Basic Expense Reduction

"Reason must govern appetite."
—Cicero

You may not know your enemies in the beginning.

At first, weight is relatively easy to lose. A moderate reduction in food intake, a moderate increase in energy expended—and those first few pounds seem to disappear overnight. Because initial weight loss is so easy, you may not be able to identify clearly the factors that contributed to weight gain. You are in the honeymoon phase of a new management job when everything responds to your slightest direction.

Eventually the pounds will come off more slowly. You will learn who your enemies really are; and you will probably discover sugar, salt, and fat lead the list.

I didn't begin to understand what I could and couldn't do until I had reached the stage where the pounds were coming off very slowly. One week I lost 37/100 of a pound, another week 12/100 of a pound. When the margin is this small, the measurements this precise, salt, fat, or sugar determined whether I lost, remained in place, or gained a fraction of a pound. I could see their impact quite clearly.

Cutting back on sugar, salt, and fats is the most basic form of weight-management expense reduction. But sometimes those expenses are hidden. When they are, you may be "spending" without knowing it. For example, most canned, processed, packaged, convenience, and fast foods, including vegetables, contain sugar and salt. Snack foods are very high in sodium. If you don't know these ingredients are part of the package, your enemies are hidden from view.

Perhaps you have reached a plateau in weight loss. You can't understand why you aren't losing. The hidden enemies may be responsible. Would you allow an unchecked cash drain to put your company at risk—or would you audit each department, seeking the source of uncharted cash flow, and dam it?

Salt has become such a key element of the American diet that its presence in food often goes undetected. Like a corporate spy posing as a trusted employee, it is a formidable enemy indeed.

You probably know that salt is responsible for water retention and that excess fluid build-up contributes to hypertension and kidney disease. Water retention also influences body weight.

Water weight is stored in tissues around the stomach, those soft and spongy rolls. It bloats ankles and swells fingers. Water weight is *weight,* but it isn't fat. Excess fat is carried in fat cells, not in fluids. Fad diets that promote instant weight loss are merely reducing fluids or, in other words, taking the water weight off.

I have learned that curtailing my salt intake promotes weight loss. But I also know that a salt intake below "normal" levels could leave me dehydrated. Salt does have a function in our diets: to retain enough water to maintain the body fluids so blood is the right consistency and tissues have the fluids they require to stay healthy. We need some

salt every day to replenish what we lose through perspiration.

But most Americans consume far more salt than they
need to fulfill this function.

Excess salt makes us thirsty and sometimes we confuse
the thirst with hunger and we eat. Salt promotes the consumption of liquids, some of them caloric, and of foods.
We need to know our bodies very well to know when we
have consumed more salt than we require in order to
function. Keeping my notebook has given me this kind
of knowledge about myself.

I know when my salt intake is in balance and when it
is not. I can see the results of too much consumption
reflected in the bottom line almost immediately. My enemy
is never hidden from view.

People who have medical problems related to salt intake can also tell when they have consumed too much salt
by increased heart rate or headaches resulting from fluids
pressing on brain tissue. Salt plays a major role in hypertension, often called the "hidden disease," from which
twenty-five million Americans suffer. Premenstrual or
menopausal women can reduce symptoms of discomfort
in part by reducing salt intake.

Thus salt is clearly a major factor in weight, and health,
management.

If you think you can control salt intake simply by passing up the salt shaker, you are wrong. You can no more
do that than you can control a company budget by monitoring one department. Diuretics are also not the answer.
People who take them regularly risk becoming dependent
on them—and/or suffering kidney impairment. Diuretics
can also cause potassium deficiency, resulting in dizziness,
nausea, and constipation.

Medical authorities advised me to check the sodium
content of the foods I eat. When I began reading labels,

I discovered the hidden costs, the ones that could clearly be eliminated without hurting the body's efficiency. I don't need canned vegetables packed in salt and sugar, so I don't eat them anymore.

Sometimes the hidden enemy is sugar, an enemy that is too often lurking in the same containers as salt.

Whereas some natural sugar is essential to provide the body with energy, we don't need nearly as much of it as our diets usually contain. We have two problems with sugar. Like salt, it is hidden in many of the foods we eat, places where we least expect it. Only a strict cost accounting, a reading of ingredient lists, discloses its presence, because we are used to its sweet taste in so many foods.

The other problem is our misconception about sugar.

Most of us believe we get a quick energy fix from sugar; and we believe this is a positive benefit, one we should enjoy when we need a fresh surge of energy during the day. We do feel peppy as sugar rushes into the bloodstream; so we think a candy bar is high-energy food. We grab one from the vending machine on the way to an important meeting.

An hour later we feel let down, irritable, exhausted, even nauseated; and we probably don't blame the feelings on the candy bar, our "energy" food. In truth, the sugar overstimulated the body's production of sugar, thus producing a low blood sugar level an hour after consumption.

Sugar is least harmful to us when we eat protein with a sugar. Because the protein is digested more slowly, it helps keep sugar from being absorbed too rapidly into the bloodstream. That's why sugar in the form of dessert may be less harmful than a sugar snack.

Some studies have indicated that a high-sugar diet contributes to performance problems on the job and lowered productivity in the workplace. Would any good manager purposely abuse or overuse sugar if he understood this?

Once you understand the real costs of sugar consumption—and you see those costs clearly reflected in the numbers recorded in your notebook—you will probably decide to reduce sugar intake.

The third hidden cost is fat, which is probably the most visible of the three enemies. We recognize on sight the high fat content of oils, butter and margarine, mayonnaise, and nuts. We may be fooled by cuts of meat that look lean and by some cheeses, which are higher in fat than many suspect. But though fat is largely visible, it is insidious in quite another way.

Fat leaves the stomach more slowly than other food constituents. Because it can't reach the bloodstream without passing through the small intestines, fat is digested slowly. This slow digestion process fools the brain. It doesn't know how much you have eaten, so it thinks you are still hungry. The brain does not receive its usual signal to shut down the appetite until the body is past "full" because the fats are moving so slowly through the system.

As a manager, you know what this means: You can't depend on the automatic chain of command to manage fat consumption. The subordinate structure can't handle this task. *You* must take control. You cannot afford to consume fats mindlessly, without managing, waiting for the tardy signal.

Yet fat is not an enemy without its uses either. One of the three necessary nutrients (along with carbohydrates and protein), fat carries the fat-soluble vitamins A, D, and E throughout the body. Keep in mind, however, some enemies are less threatening than others: Unsaturated fats found in liquid oils and vegetable products are thought to be preferable to saturated fats found in meats and hard oils such as butter.

But fat in excess quantities, whether saturated or not, still contributes to cholesterol and triglyceride problems.

Although no *direct* evidence links cholesterol and heart disease, much indirect evidence indicates excessive fat consumption is a contributor to heart disease. Cholesterol is present in every cell of the body; and its presence is necessary. The body will make cholesterol out of other substances if you don't take in sufficient quantities.

Yet an excess of cholesterol circulating in the bloodstream creates waxy deposits, which injure blood vessel walls and clog arteries. When the blockages are large enough, obstructing artery channels, a stroke or heart attack can result.

Triglycerides are the fats visible in foods and the main component of our own fat tissues. Those calories consumed in a meal and not used immediately by tissues are converted to triglycerides before being sent to the fat cells for storage. Release of triglycerides from fat tissue is controlled by hormones to meet the body's energy needs between meals. Many medical authorities believe that some people with an excess amount of triglycerides in their blood plasma are at greater risk of coronary disease.

What I learned about the hidden costs of sugar, salt, and fats—and the costs of another potential enemy, alcohol, which is rich in calories and low in nutrients—helped me to reduce those expenses in my weight-management budget. I began to analyze the expenses in the same way I would analyze all the expenses involved in a construction project. Through the Strategic Weight-Control System, I became able to control the hidden costs. By accurately measuring my weight each day, I could also measure the impact of sugar, salt, and fats.

Without this system, I might be able to identify my enemies, but I would never be able to gauge their effect with this degree of accuracy.

13

Synergy of Mind and Body

"The only way to create more of the enzymes
needed to metabolize fat is through exercise."
—Jane Fonda

We haven't talked yet in detail about the third component in weight management: energy expenditure.

Some people view an exercise program with as much
enthusiasm as they do a tax audit. But I believe exercise
is essential to weight management. Trying to manage your
weight by focusing only on the amounts and types of food
consumed is certainly possible, but it's more difficult because you are working with two variables rather than
three.

Also, if you diet without exercise, you may lose as much
lean muscle tissue as fat. Muscle loss decreases your ability
to burn fat. Thus it will be harder for you to maintain
that weight loss than it will be for the person who exercises.

By increasing energy expenditure, you can lose more
quickly or you can choose to eat more food and still maintain a desirable weight. How you balance the equation
depends on you. If the success of the equation depends
on all three elements, you will have a greater margin in
which to manipulate.

Managing weight without exercise is like running a company on a short staff. It's possible of course, if everybody works overtime. But do you really want to work overtime for the rest of your life?

The problem most of us have with exercise is overcoming the psychological barrier: We would rather take an elevator than walk six flights of stairs. In a sense, exercise is contrary to the modern concept of progress in America. Our technological advances in the past century have been geared toward limiting the physical effort required in one's daily work life. We have given more and more of our work to machines—and been glad to do so. Only in the past decade has exercise come back into style.

Before I tell you to exercise, we need a good definition of that term. I do not want you to be left with another one of those words like *thinner, happy, successful.* So what do we mean by *exercise?*

Some authorities maintain that exercise is aerobic activity. (The word *aerobic* means promoting the supply of oxygen.) They refer to the pulse-rate system of exercise developed by Dr. Kenneth Cooper, which involves moving vigorously and steadily (running, jogging, dancing, etc.) for a period of twenty to forty-five minutes, three to five times a week, so the cardiovascular system (heart, lungs, and circulatory system) works at a rate that demands large amounts of oxygen.

Exercise gurus believe anything less "doesn't count."

They remind me of the time-and-motion theorists, "efficiency experts," once hired by companies to measure and analyze every step involved in a specific job and then assign a time to each task. Supposedly the experts could make employees work as efficiently as machines. This was called a "science."

Obviously it wasn't.

Today fitness gurus treat exercise in the same way.

According to the tenets of their "science," you aren't getting real benefits unless you choose a certain type of activity, work at a given intensity, for a specified duration of time and frequency.

That's why exercise scares so many of us. We think we have to apply this rigid formula to our lives. If we aren't ready to take up marathon running, we feel there is no place for us in the exercise ethic.

I have chosen to define exercise very simply as *energy expended*.

Yes, you are going to expend more energy in an hour of aerobic dancing than you will by walking an extra block a day. But walking that extra block is better than not walking it, and walking it will probably encourage you to expend additional energy in other areas of your life.

When I began to work with the Strategic Weight-Control System, I knew I would have to increase energy expenditure, but I didn't know how. Medical authorities caution against taking up strenuous exercise suddenly, and especially in midlife. The person who is twenty pounds overweight and gets out of breath climbing one flight of stairs cannot put on a jogging suit and run for a mile or two. Even making the attempt is hazardous.

I began to make very small changes in the way I expended energy. I took the stairs rather than the elevator. My office at HBE is on the sixth floor, so several times a day I walked up and down those stairs.

I stopped looking for the most convenient parking places when I went out. On business trips I built as much walking as possible into the day's activities. Gradually I increased the amounts of time and distance I could walk. Then I began to expend energy in forms more commonly regarded as exercise. Now my bedroom looks like a small gym; it houses a stationary bike and various weights.

Once I began to increase my level of physical activity,

I knew just how much I had been kidding myself all those years about feeling "good." Today I honestly do feel good, thanks in large part to exercise, which has many benefits beyond calorie burning. Exercise enhances your sense of well-being. The more you do, the more you want to do. It could be compared to making money on good investments. The rewards are that tangible.

They are also well documented. The U.S. Public Health Service, the government's top health agency, recently released a report saying, "Based on evidence, physical fitness and exercise is one of the 15 areas of greatest importance for improving the health of the public." Moderate levels of exercise reduce the risks of coronary disease and obesity, as well as reduce the symptoms of depression and anxiety.

Maybe you're impressed with the benefits but a little skeptical about how they can be achieved. Once you understand how exercise works, you will probably want to increase your own energy expenditure levels too.

There is only one way fat can be removed from fat cells: by transference to muscle cells, where it is burned for energy. Remember those storage closets backlogged with supplies of fat? The supplies can't get out of the closets without purchase orders originating in the muscle cells.

You can lose weight by dramatically cutting calorie intake, but it's hard to sustain this weight loss without increasing exercise. We have learned that the body adjusts its set point to accommodate the lower calorie levels. We know the body can run very efficiently, using as little fat as possible, to protect its fat stores, if we don't force it to work harder and use fat *effectively*, rather than *efficiently*.

But your body has a hard time stockpiling its fat supplies if you are exercising regularly. Even moderate exercise increases the metabolic rate and sends the order down for fat. The residual effects of exercise may keep the metabolic rate higher for hours following exercise.

Exercise also increases muscle mass, which means more cells will be ordering fat. The body needs more calories simply to maintain lean muscle mass than to maintain fat cells. As you exercise and build muscle mass, the more fat you will burn, simply standing still.

Exercise also promotes the production of more enzymes for burning fat. The enzymes speed the conduction of the fat particle into the muscle, where it can be burned. A fat person who does not exercise has fewer enzymes for fat metabolism so that any physical activity he undertakes is less productive in terms of fat burning than the same kind and amount of activity undertaken by a person with greater muscle mass.

So exercise is like a good credit rating: It keeps expanding your management potential.

When I understood the cumulative effects of exercise, I was excited. At last I had the knowledge of all three components I needed to run my body as successfully as I ran my company. I could understand all the forces that affected my weight each day. Once I understood them, I could manage my weight.

Some members of the Control Group Team were already convinced of the importance of exercise before they began the program. Others became believers as they learned more. And some few still hold out, refusing to exercise.

One woman, who maintains her weight through the method of continuous accountability, insists she would rather starve to death than exercise.

I can't emphasize enough that the Strategic Weight-Control System gives you the freedom to make those choices, *any* choices. But look at the facts closely before you choose. We manage by making and implementing decisions, but we can't make those decisions without having all the facts.

Understand what exercise is and what it does for you before you slight the energy-expended portion of your equation.

When I listen to people tell me they are able to maintain their weight by stringently controlling two of the three areas, I don't feel comfortable about the way they are choosing to manage. They can do it this way, but will it be the best management practice for long-term, sustained results? A management approach that deals separately with each department and doesn't constantly coordinate the activities of all the departments leads to duplication of effort, wasted time, monetary loss.

My estimating people want to estimate; my building people want to build. It's up to me to coordinate their efforts, to make sure each is working toward the overall corporate goals.

A weight-management approach that doesn't coordinate and balance the three functions—amount and kinds of food and energy expended—could waste time, energy, and money.

When I look at the numbers in my notebook, I am trying to understand myself, to understand exactly how each of those three forces affects me each day. I am not merely interested in seeing what I weigh.

14

Performance Review III

"A man who has to win every battle is asking the impossible of himself and the world, and is likely to collapse the first time he encounters defeat."
—from *Power,* by Michael Korda

Q. I take diuretics daily, as prescribed by my doctor. Would I have to take those diuretics even if I lost weight?

A. Would you need to hire temporary staff for an overflow of work if the overflow didn't exist?

My medical authorities tell me the overwhelming majority of Americans on diuretics are overweight—and would not have to take this medication if they lost weight. Exercise, by the way, in addition to being a good method of weight reduction, is also a means of helping the body eliminate excess fluids naturally through perspiration.

Q. When I am nervous or anxious, I crave salty snacks. When I am depressed, I crave sugar. These are, and always have been, my dietary downfalls. How can the system help me change that?

A. These are short-term solutions for long-term problems—and like many stopgap measures, they are expensive. Think of curtailing salt, fats, and sugar as an exercise in quality control. Quality control is nothing more than controlling the downside by deciding how many defects are acceptable. *You* decide what is an acceptable amount of these expense items in your management budget. Once you have set your standards, maintain them.

Some medical evidence indicates that hypertensive people have a higher threshold for salt. They may require larger quantities of salt before their taste buds register saltiness. And some evidence exists that sugar, especially sugar in conjunction with chocolate, does release a chemical in the brain that elevates our mood for a while.

Now that you understand how these desires work, you can manage them.

Using the Strategic Weight-Control System can help you abandon stopgap measures. You will see the effects of these choices in numerical terms. You won't be able to kid yourself about their impact anymore. This will help you change the snacking habits you know are bad for you.

Q. I am very confused about fats. Some fat is necessary, even good for you, but too much fat is bad. I've read that some fats are better than others. Why? And which?

A. Paid holidays are "good" for all of us, aren't they? They give us a breather from routine, a chance to replenish our energy and enthusiasm. But an excess of paid holidays would hurt productivity—and company profits.

Consider fats a paid holiday.

The "good" fats, polyunsaturated and monounsaturated fats, have proven to be cholesterol reducers. They lower the levels of "bad" cholesterol, low density lipoproteins (LDL), which is thought to be associated with heart disease. Polyunsaturated fats also lower the levels of "good" cholesterol, high density lipoproteins (HDL), thought to protect the body from heart attacks. Monounsaturated fats don't lower HDL levels.

Among the good monounsaturates is olive oil.

Q. Is there a perfect exercise, one that will provide cardiovascular benefits as well as tone, strengthen, increase flexibility—and burn calories?

A. Is there a perfect approach to management, one theory any manager can use in any situation? No. So it is with exercise.

Walking is considered by many to be a *near* ideal exercise. Anyone can walk. It's inexpensive: No special clothing or equipment is required. Walking is safe; there is little potential for strained muscles or other injuries. And brisk walking will give you most of the benefits you seek.

But what if you don't like to walk? You won't make yourself walk for long if you hate it. Maybe you would enjoy something else instead. What if I insisted walking was the "perfect" exercise? Would that change your mind? I doubt it.

Q. I exercise vigorously once a week for more than an hour. People tell me this isn't enough, that I am wasting my time. Am I?

A. If you are running or indulging in other vigorous exercise once a week for an hour or more you are risking injury and, depending on your age, possibly increasing the chances of having a stroke. Would you let a new employee represent your company at an important conference? Don't force your body into rigorous performance conditions on a weekly basis either. It isn't prepared for the effort.

Walking for fifteen minutes a day, or increasing energy expenditure in a similarly moderate but regular fashion, is preferable. In the long run, it will provide more benefits and less risk.

Q. You say even a moderate increase in energy expenditure is beneficial. But isn't it true that you don't get full cardiovascular benefits unless you work out vigorously, elevating the heart rate, at least three times a week?

A. Would you ask me this question: Isn't it true that only a company that grosses in excess of $100 million a year is truly profitable and that a company grossing less is not getting any benefits from its profits?

A recent study conducted jointly by Harvard and Stanford universities on seventeen thousand men found a lower death rate and other preventative health benefits were obtained from *moderate* levels of exercise, levels far below the fevered pitch most fitness gurus recommend. The men with the fewest problems were those who had regular habits of walking and climbing stairs, who played sports such as golf or tennis, but who were not long-distance runners, weight lifters, etc.

Evidence indicates that those who exercise excessively, such as joggers who exceed fifteen miles a week, are at high risk for injuries to bones and joints.

Q. I have seen those charts telling how many calories you burn for each exercise. For example, you have to run eight minutes to burn only one hundred calories. And you have to burn thirty-five hundred calories to lose only one pound of fat. I don't see how exercise can help that much. Wouldn't I have to exercise a lot to lose weight?

A. Those numbers are misleading. Looking at them to gauge the calorie-burning effects of exercise is like trying to evaluate a corporation's overall profit picture by studying one small division.

In addition to burning a specific number of calories, exercise increases the metabolic rate, which in turn helps you burn more calories during normal activity or even when at rest than you would have burned without the exercise. And exercise also increases the secretion of enzymes that burn fat and enlarges muscle mass, which burns more calories than fatty tissue does. The number of calories actually burned by exercise is far greater than the figures on any chart will lead you to believe.

Q. How do I know if I'm eating properly and working out enough? Is there a way of measuring fitness?

A. There are many "tests" you can take to measure fitness. They are often printed in newspapers and magazines in the form of quizzes—like those quizzes that supposedly help you measure your management skills. If you want to take them, you can. To be absolutely sure of good general health, you need regular physicals, as recommended by your doctor.

But if you are looking for a quick answer to the question "Am I fit?" turn the question around and ask yourself if you are successfully managing your weight. Medical authorities say the first requirement for fitness is maintaining proper weight.

Q. I am afraid if I exercise my appetite will increase. And then I will undo the good I am doing by dieting. Isn't that likely to happen?

A. No. If anything, exercise actually decreases the appetite. This myth, which many use as an excuse for remaining sedentary, reminds me of office gossip. How often is a hot rumor really true? And how often do people use gossip and innuendo as an excuse to make a decision they shouldn't make?

Q. I want to find the right exercise to help me spot-reduce. How can I do that?

A. There is no such thing as spot-reducing. If you had to cut expenditures in your budget, you could, for example, cut your electric bill by turning down the thermostat or closing off a room—but you couldn't cut that bill by deciding to spot-reduce the temperature in one room to sixty, in another to fifty, unless you have individual thermostats in each room of the house.

You can do exercises such as sit-ups or push-ups to tone the muscles under the fat. Thus you may look leaner in those places. But you cannot actually regulate where the fat will come off by spot-reducing exercises.

Exercise reduces us by cutting the amount of fat in our fat cells. The body's regulator decides which fat cells give up their stores first. "Spot-reducing" on demand isn't possible.

Q. When I go to the spa, I lose weight. Why does it come right back on the next day?

A. You haven't lost fat, but rather water weight. The belief that fat can be sweated out is another one of those hot rumors, not founded in truth.

15

Management Stress

"If you have a job without aggravations, you
don't have a job."
— Malcolm Forbes

A successful manager *must* be able to manage under
stress.

Managing under stress obviously requires more skill
and coordination than managing when everything is going
smoothly. But we kid ourselves about workplace stress:
We like to think of those easy, relatively stress-free days
as "normal," when in fact they are not. Most days we must
manage under some degree of stress. At HBE, "normal"
is fairly hectic; and I imagine this is true at any other
successful company.

If, as a weight manager, you give yourself license *not*
to manage under stress, you will find yourself not managing a good percentage of the time.

Even after I had examined nutritional and exercise
data and understood the dynamics of how food and energy expenditure affect my bottom line, I was still tempted
at times to behave in the typically destructive stress-
response pattern—to eat more and exercise less. I certainly was not alone. Medical authorities tell me that stress

is the most common cause of overeating and thus the most serious threat to strategic weight management.

Some people respond to stress by losing their appetites. Unfortunately, most of us respond to stress by eating more. We don't really enjoy the food we consume then; we just eat it.

I knew what would happen to my management program if I gave in to stress. Monitoring the bottom line helped me keep that habit in check.

Several members of the control group also reported that their significant weight-management problems occurred in times of stress. One said, "When I am pushed with a heavy deadline, I don't take the time to eat right. Instead of balanced meals, I eat a lot of high-calorie fast foods and snacks; and I don't exercise either."

Another told me, "While I'm under the gun, I'm okay. When the pressure is over, I eat. After I've been through a particular crisis, maybe working on a project where deadlines were nearly impossible to meet because of factors outside my control, like the weather or supply shortages or labor problems, I reward myself by letting down. Food is part of the letting down. I feel like I've gone through so much I owe myself indulgence."

So we use food as a coping mechanism—even though the mechanism doesn't work. On the job we would not continue to use a management technique that time and again had failed to accomplish our objectives, would we?

Kaye's use of this mechanism is typical. She said, "In the past, I bought myself an ice cream sundae on the way home from work whenever I'd had a rough day. Well, I have always felt miserable about eating that sundae even as I was putting the last spoonful into my mouth. Why did I do it? What was the point when it made me feel worse, not better?"

Monitoring the bottom line helped her recognize that habit and break it. Now she has an ice cream sundae only when she really wants one, not in response to a mindless compulsion.

There is a big difference between eating because you have a taste for it—because you really want that ice cream—and using the food as a comforting buffer between you and management stress.

Now that you are using the Strategic Weight-Control System, you too are becoming aware of how *every* choice made affects the bottom line. You have probably identified the stress eating habit in your own management style. The system gives you the method of controlling that habit, but you must use it as directed.

A few of the Control Group Team members said initially they "forgot" or "were too busy" to weigh themselves on the days when they felt most under stress. Fortunately, they recognized that skipping the weighing process because of stress is not acceptable. This situation is not comparable to that of the business traveler who cannot find a scale while out of town.

"I forgot" or "I was too busy" are excuses, not reasons. When the team members stopped making those excuses, they began to manage under stress. If you can't manage under stress, you can't manage.

Studies have shown that obese people far more often than people of normal weight use eating when under stress as a coping response. They increase their food intake whenever they feel anxious or tense. Consuming food under such conditions isn't a pleasurable experience. Often they barely taste what they eat.

Eating when under stress is an unconscious response. The more you allow this response to control you, the more you will probably weigh. We can only control the response if we are aware of what it is doing to us, if we are holding ourselves constantly accountable for the bottom line.

It also has helped me, as I am sure it will help you, to understand the physiology of the stress response.

Stress triggers hormonal and metabolic changes in the body, which shouldn't surprise us. We know how a stressful office situation triggers a reaction from us. In a crisis situation, people visibly gear up to meet the increased demands on their time, energy, skills.

Similarly, in crisis, the body gears up in its own way—in part by asking for more food than it needs. What we interpret as hunger during those crisis times may actually be an inner discomfort that we try to soothe, a void we attempt to fill with food.

Eating actually does help minimize some of the effects of stress on the body, just as letting off steam in the office may reduce stress. The parasympathetic nervous system is activated during digestion, producing that relaxed feeling one has after a good meal. However, when you have eaten foods you didn't want to eat, you have lost control. And the unhappiness you feel about losing control soon destroys the good feeling of relaxation. This is not unlike the feeling you might have after losing your temper in front of a client, a superior, or a colleague whose respect you desire. You wish you had remained in control, don't you?

Control is the key. As I have said before, I don't believe in diets, in denying yourself the foods you really want. Using the Strategic Weight-Control System, you can eat the foods you like, enjoy restaurant meals and social evenings with friends. You don't have to diet. I don't.

But eating when under stress isn't pleasurable. It has to do with mindless compulsion, not desire—with being managed, not managing. You don't make a conscious choice to enjoy a good meal. Instead you respond to an unconscious coping mechanism that was first programmed into you as a baby, when your mother stopped your tears with a cookie.

Now you understand the stress-eating response. Understanding it and having the tool to control it will change your management pattern. You will no longer find yourself sitting at a desk looking down at the remains of a sweet snack you can't even remember tasting, regretting the consumption of this and so many such snacks in the past. Though we usually do turn to calorie-laden and often sweet foods to alleviate stress, we seldom enjoy the actual consumption of them.

As soon as I became aware of my food intake, I stopped using food as a stress reliever. When you aren't constantly aware, you eat in such an automatic fashion that you lie to yourself about how much you have eaten. You have no realization of the size of the lie either. When you barely taste, and certainly don't enjoy, much of the food you consume, it's very easy to misrepresent the amount.

When people tell me they don't understand *why* they're fat because they "don't eat that much," I know they aren't exactly lying. Because they are using food to relieve stress and because they have been doing it for so long, they have lost track of how much they eat. When they have no reliable means of measurement, they have no means to change.

Once the Control Group Team members identified the stress-eating syndrome, they were able to manage it. Each found alternative means of coping with stress. So can you.

If you were supervising an employee who always responded to a work overload by nonproductive panic, you would sit the employee down, explain the situation, show him what he's doing wrong, and help him find some better means of coping. Similarly, you may have to offer yourself a coping mechanism to replace eating to relieve stress.

Obviously, the choice of the method will be an individual decision. The Strategic Weight-Control System is developed as a tool for self-management, not a system to manage you.

Some of the Control Group Team members feel the gratification of eating is necessary during periods of stress, so they replace high-calorie snacks with diet soda or raw vegetables. Others find that exercise works well to alleviate stress, so they take lunchtime walks. And all of us have found we are much better at solving the office problems that cause stress when we aren't turning mindlessly to food to dull that stress. We put our energies into problem solving, force ourselves to deal head-on with our problems. We must manage when we cannot retreat.

According to medical authorities, you will be less susceptible to the temptation of the stress-eating response if you have good nutritional habits and exercise regularly. Poor dietary habits and a sedentary life-style contribute to anxiousness, irritability, failure to cope successfully with stress. These habits can impair your ability to meet management demands effectively.

Again, once you understand the numbers you're writing in that notebook each day, the bare bones of your weight-management program, you will be better able to manage. No surprises will catch you off guard. You will be prepared for every management situation, including stress.

Without the Strategic Weight-Control System, stress usually catches us by surprise. Our body perceives stress as a threat and responds by requesting more food, either in a short-lived burst of high-calorie snacking or in prolonged periods of overeating that can last for days or weeks. But we can intervene in that process. We can *manage*.

Good managers are never surprised by crisis situations because they have anticipated each crisis that could possibly occur. They will not accept excuses or rationalizations for why the job wasn't done—not from themselves or from subordinates. When you stop accepting the excuse "I was under a lot of pressure," you will short-circuit the stress-eating response. You will be able to override the body's computer.

16

The Roadblocks to Self-Management

"The discipline of desire is the background of character."

—John Locke

What interests me about weight-management roadblocks is how they are constructed: We put them in our own paths.

The barriers to management success put in the road by other people or external forces can be negotiated so much more easily than our own roadblocks. We study them and find a path around them. We pick them up and move them aside.

In the business of constructing hospitals and hotels, for example, we are frequently faced with delays in shipments of materials, a labor force that varies in skill and cost from one job site to another, labor laws and building codes that differ widely from city to city and state to state. Building a first-quality hotel or hospital within a given time period is a challenge. We know from the beginning a certain number of barriers will be a part of the course that must be negotiated. We anticipate them, sometimes with zest. What good manager doesn't like a challenge?

The roadblocks we put in our paths, however, are much harder to get around. We are fighting ourselves, not external forces. And we have to understand ourselves very well to wage this battle and win.

The Strategic Weight-Control System has helped me to do this. And it can help you too. Those numbers are more than mere numbers. They are symbols with their own meanings in relation to each other. They are more complex, far more meaningful, than I imagined they would be.

When I look at my entries, I can trace my eating and exercise patterns with an acute degree of accuracy. I know when I ate and what and why—and how it affected the bottom line. I have begun to understand *all* the factors motivating me to eat or not to eat, to exercise or to remain sedentary. Through this understanding, I have gained control.

Since I am in control of all those factors, I am also in control of my weight.

You know how critical numbers are to a business. Profit statements tell you more than how much money a company made or lost. They tell you where the company made or lost that money—and how it did—and why. The numbers are symbols. A close reading of them provides a detailed account of that company's life.

You can read your own life in the same way in the numbers you record in your notebook.

You will see your own roadblocks reflected clearly in those numbers. And you will be able to deal with the roadblocks because you do see them now. Before I began managing my weight, I ignored the existence of road-blocks.

I grew up, as you probably did, believing that cleaning my plate was a virtue. When I was young, fat babies were considered "healthy" babies. Fat was supposed to protect us, provide us with warmth in the winter and strength in case of illness.

The first roadblock to weight management most of us

have to overcome is this early training. We have to learn that it is better to leave the leftovers on our plates than put them on our waistlines. We must recognize that fat is unhealthy, so unhealthy it has been declared a disease.

I was out with my wife the other night when we decided on the spur of the moment to have a pizza. We split a small pizza; and we didn't even finish that. It wasn't a particularly good pizza; and a little of it was enough to satisfy our taste for pizza. Before I began using the Strategic Weight-Control System, I would have finished that pizza—not because I was hungry, not because it was good, only because it was there.

Most members of the Control Group Team, whether in their twenties or fifty-plus, have reported the same problems with early conditioning. Most mothers reward good behavior with candy, soothe tears with cookies or ice cream, insist children clean their plates. In many of their childhood homes, food was also a source of ethnic pride; and ethnic menus don't include diet foods. In these families, food is equated with love. Eating is tied into being a good son or daughter.

One man told me, "I have always felt like I made my mother look bad if I refused her food. I'm over forty, and I still feel guilty if I don't eat anything when I visit her. She's spent her whole life being a good cook. If I don't eat her food, I'm telling her she wasted her life."

For most of us, family social life still revolves around food, even if our mothers have jobs and are not known as "cooks." Attend a family reunion and everyone will push a favorite dish at you. Weddings and birthdays, holiday meals, all the red-letter family occasions are marked by overeating. Thanksgiving is a holiday, in fact, that is devoted entirely to stuffing—ourselves, not merely the turkeys.

If we let other people push food on us, food we don't

want or need, we are being managed. We are not just being managed, we are being pushed around. Would we let anyone treat us this way on the job?

Many of the Control Group Team, particularly the women, also identified another roadblock in their paths to successful weight management. They felt they had learned to "use" fat as an issue in power struggles. Maybe they had parents who wanted them to be slim children; they rebelled by being fat. Maybe they had husbands who wanted thin wives; they used fat as a way of settling other scores in the marriage. Or maybe they got fat because their mothers had; being thin seemed like a rejection of mother's life and values.

We've all seen managers function on this management level, haven't we? Consider this typical scenario: *I know you need my report by Monday if you're going to finish your work on time, but the truth is I don't want you to finish your work on time. I can hold you back if I procrastinate.* That's interdepartmental sabotage, something that happens often in some companies, only occasionally in others. A good manager spots this practice immediately and squelches it.

A weight manager who allows psychological roadblocks to prevent him or her from successfully managing is allowing one department to sabotage another. Don't let that happen. Identify your roadblocks and tear them down.

"Maybe I stay fat because deep down I'm afraid of being too attractive," one young woman told me. "I am not sure if I can deal with everything our culture expects of an attractive young woman. I am not sure if I can be good in business and be other things too. This way I don't have to try."

Once she had recognized her own form of interdepartmental sabotage, she began to eliminate it.

But she only understood this much about herself *after* she'd put the Strategic Weight-Control System to work in her life. By working with the numbers, she was forced to admit that much of her snacking was a reaction to a psychological, not a physical, need. She could see clearly on her chart where she had binged and she made herself admit why.

We have talked a great deal about controlling all three elements of the weight equation—amount and kinds of foods, and energy expended. Yet we really can't manage those elements effectively if we allow roadblocks to stand in our way. It's probably not possible to make progress without first demolishing your own roadblocks.

There are many definitions of productivity in business, but a good one should take into account the organization as a whole, all the efforts that influence performance, not just the amount of work an employee or groups of employees can do. The work, how well it is performed, and how well that performance meets the overall objectives of the company determine the productivity numbers. If there are roadblocks to productivity within a company, they can be discovered in an insightful reading of the numbers.

Weight management is no different. Productivity in weight management can be measured by how well you integrate the elements to achieve success, the bottom-line weight you want to maintain. Just as the profitable, productive company is well managed, so is the profitable, productive weight-control program. Those roadblocks are the last obstacle in your way—in the way of good management and good productivity numbers.

Managers who come from families where fat is acceptable, even preferable, may find it difficult to eliminate those roadblocks. According to some folklore, fat is "happy." And worse, in some families, the person who is not fat is made to feel guilty, a traitor to the family ethic. The others resent his thinness, his success at weight management. If you come from such a family, you will have to work against it.

A very successful manager is often resented by others, even his closest colleagues, because of his outstanding success.

The overweight spouse or sister, coworker or friend, may resent your success as you become an Effective Weight Manager. People who aren't managing their own weight often attempt to pull others down to their level of non-achievement. They are threatened by your success, by your new independence. While they are slaves to fat cells and set points, manipulated by circumstances, and stalled at roadblocks, *you* are free, freed by the numbers. No wonder they are jealous.

How many times have you seen the workplace status quo upset by a promotion?

When one person is promoted over a group of peers, especially peers with whom he or she has been close, an uncomfortable situation can result. The skilled new manager copes with the discomfort. He does what he can to help others adjust to the change in his status, but he certainly doesn't throw away his new promotion because it threatens others.

Unfortunately, a surprising number of people who have lost weight do throw success away, by regaining the weight lost, encouraged in part by overweight friends and relatives who would rather see the manager fail than admit success is possible.

In contrast to these heavy psychological roadblocks, some of the obstacles we throw in our own paths seem like minor ones. They focus on one aspect of the weight equation. Or perhaps they are motivated by laziness or the simple reluctance to change habits, patterns.

Such roadblocks include familiar excuses: "It's too much trouble to cook a diet meal for myself and regular food for the family"; "Diet food is so expensive"; "Diet meals are so monotonous"; "I don't have time to exercise"; "Exercise is just so boring."

Without the Strategic Weight-Control System, those roadblocks assume larger porportions than they should. It is possible for us to keep kidding ourselves about our weight because we are used to losing weight, then being stalled at these familiar points. We let our past failures set us up for future failures. In short, we behave like the least valued employee, rather than managers. No one is really in charge.

Within the system, those roadblocks are reduced, defined by the numbers, outlined clearly so we can eliminate them. We see them for what they are: barriers that can be removed, not permanent parts of the road.

17

The Flexible Manager

"A dinner lubricates business."
—James Boswell

I travel frequently—so often that I can remember few weeks in recent years when I've spent every day in Saint Louis. There were probably *no* weeks when I didn't consume several meals away from home. Thus I eat a great many restaurant meals either while traveling or in town conducting business or socializing. Like you, I am accustomed to cementing professional and personal alliances over a table filled with food and drink.

If I couldn't manage my weight while traveling or dining out, I wouldn't be able to manage at all. The same is probably true for you. If you have decided managing away from your own table is not possible, then you have decided *managing* is not possible.

A good manager is flexible, able to cope with conditions outside the realm of the usual, able to function on his own corporate turf or someone else's. You would never say, "I'm sorry I can't do business out of town. You'll have to come to my office in my city or we can't make a deal." You would be flexible and travel where you had to travel to get the job done.

Similarly, if you are going to be a successful weight manager, you will have to be flexible. You may travel a lot or dine in restaurants often. A peripatetic life is common now and no excuse for losing track.

A dozen years ago most business people felt pressured to indulge in a heavy lunch, usually a two-martini lunch, as a prelude to a business deal. In the mid-eighties, when so many people are weight and health conscious, none of us has to feel out of place ordering a lighter fare and drinking a glass of wine or bottled water or club soda in place of a cocktail. Granted, I still would not feel entirely comfortable ordering a salad with no dressing while dining with a group of heavy eaters, but then I don't have to do that to keep my weight under control. My choices don't have to be that drastic because they are balanced carefully through this system of continuous accountability.

I do order more fish, chicken, and seafood, more broiled and baked entrees, and eat less beef and pork, less fried foods and those covered in heavy sauces, less bread and butter and desserts. If I am satisfied with a few bites of bread or dessert, I leave the rest on my plate. And I don't carry anything home or back to the hotel in a carry-out bag.

Many of HBE's employees also travel frequently, some more often than I do. Several Control Group Team members have told me that in the past their "diets" fell apart when they were on the road. Away from home and the regular routines of the office, they ate more than usual and expended less energy. Yet they excused themselves with the reassuring thought, "I can't do anything about weight when I'm traveling or eating out. It's out of my control then."

I had told myself much the same lie before I began managing my weight. It was easy and convenient to overeat while traveling. Food compensated for the inconvenience of travel, the loneliness of being away from my home and family. It was also a means of relieving fatigue at the end of the day.

Like kids on a holiday, we all used being out of town as an excuse for nonmanaging.

My own experience with the Strategic Weight-Control System—and that of other group members—has proven our past line of reasoning false. We do not have to lose control away from home. Business dining situations *can* be managed as easily as home dining, once you begin monitoring the bottom line.

Unless you are holding yourself accountable, however, the temptations to give up control are obvious. First, traveling and dining out offer a plethora of choices: so many places to eat, so many items on a menu. A salesperson on the road is often tempted to grab a sandwich "fast" rather than wait to be served a balanced lower-calorie meal. Anyone traveling alone feels the temptation to order large meals and gooey desserts from room service to assuage loneliness and compensate for the effort expended during the day. People who travel often overeat from fatigue, which they confuse with hunger.

And when you are entertaining a client out of town or in, you're certainly tempted to pull out all the stops and order every course at a restaurant. Partly you want to impress him. Partly you want to assure him he can have anything he wants since he may be taking his order cues from you.

The other built-in drawback to travel involves the rest of the weight-management equation, energy expended.

Those of us who have exercise routines at home seldom practice them on the road. We believe our schedules are too crowded. Or we can't find a gym. We're afraid to jog in strange cities. And if we practice aerobic dancing in a hotel room, won't our energetic jumping around disturb a guest on the floor below?

We have at least one "good" excuse for every day spent out of town.

Is it possible, then, to be an Effective Weight Manager while traveling and dining out, when you are confronted with so many temptations and choices, and your conscience is assuaged by so many good excuses?

I have proven it is. So have many other Control Group Team members. You can be an Effective Weight Manager anywhere by maintaining constant awareness. The Strategic Weight-Control System is simple, basic, unchanging. The only real difference between traveling and staying home is the excess of choices. You have so many more options; and you have identified fewer of them in advance.

At home, you know what the options are: The contents of the cabinets and the refrigerator; and those options may be even further limited by the time you have for food preparation. Those choices seem very limited when compared to the choices that exist in a new city, a favorite restaurant.

But the existence of a greater number of choices doesn't force you to make *bad* choices.

I plan to limit choices in advance wherever I can. For example, the foods I now stock on the company plane are different than those I used to order. I may ask for fruit and salad plates rather than the steak and baked potato I might have ordered in the past. When dining out, I prefer not to select restaurants where the menu is made up almost exclusively of rich and high-calorie foods. And I build exercise into my business trips by walking as much as possible. Where once I would have taken a cab from the hotel to a meeting or a restaurant, now I walk when possible.

And I don't hesitate to ask for specially prepared foods if I want them. Nor should you. We are paying enough money to request that a sauce be withheld from a dish, that the meat be broiled, or that the dressing be served on the side. I am surprised when people who are aggressive in business situations turn meek in restaurants. They may be served food that is unacceptable—salad soaked in dressing, fried foods thick with grease—yet they feel obligated to eat that food rather than send it back or leave it on their plates.

Nowhere is mother's training—"Clean your plate!"—more out of place than in restaurants.

As soon as you understand the real choices you have in restaurants, you will be in charge of the meals you eat in them. Until you do, the restaurant is in charge.

Now that you are using the Strategic Weight-Control System, your life need no longer be divided into periods when you actively "diet" or manage your weight and periods when you allow circumstances, including travel or dining out, to manage you. Begin treating travel and dining out as parts of your life, not lapses from real life. When you recognize the challenges these particular situations create, you are prepared to meet them.

A wide range of choices should be no more threatening to a weight manager than a business manager. If I told you that you could select one new employee from a group of ten exceptional people or from a group of two exceptional people, which would you prefer. The good choices on the road are many too. Making them should not be so difficult after all.

18

Performance Review IV

"If I believe I cannot do something, it makes me
incapable of doing it. But when I believe I can,
then I acquire the ability to do it even if I didn't
have it at the beginning. . . . "
—Mahatma Gandhi

Q. I have been using the Strategic Weight-Control System for nearly two months; and I have lost ten pounds, halfway to my goal. But this is the point where I usually fail in dieting. Thinking about losing those last ten pounds makes me nervous; and being nervous usually makes me eat. What if I fail again?

A. If you were halfway to completion of a quarterly management goal, would you worry in the same way about failure? Would you fear "losing" the gains made? Probably not. You have enough confidence in yourself as a manager to believe you will achieve your goals and certainly will not "lose" progress already made. And you understand that goals are continually updated. As a weight manager, you will have maintenance goals once you have achieved weight-loss goals.

The Strategic Weight-Control System is a management system to help you achieve those goals, not a diet. Since the system has become an integral part of your daily routine, you don't have to worry about failure as you would if you were on yet another "diet." The system forces you to keep continuous track of where you stand. It treats progress as a journey, not a destination.

Look at what you have already learned about yourself after only two months with the system: You have identified the stress-eating response. You know that you have a psychological block that has stopped you in the past from completing weight-loss goals.

As long as you continue to use the system, you will continue to learn about yourself. You cannot fail. If you were on a diet, you could fail simply by consuming more than the allotted number of calories for a day or two. The system forces you to record and analyze data. It doesn't pass judgment on the data or on you.

You interpret the data and use it to achieve your goals. I am convinced that "failure" is not possible unless you stop weighing, recording, averaging, and charting the numbers.

Q. After four weeks on the system, I am faithfully following the directions and losing weight. What worries me still is the abundance of choices I have. Since you do not give us a calorie limit or a menu plan, we are on our own. What is to stop us from making the wrong choices, especially under stress?

A. What is to stop you from making the wrong choices on the job? No management book can tell you what to do all the time. Who is to keep you on track then?

You are.

You are in charge of your weight too. As the weight manager, you are the only person who can make the choices. Using the system "faithfully" insures you will make good choices.

Q. Eating when under stress is my biggest problem.

Would you recommend some kind of stress-management training for me?

A. If you came to me with a specific management problem at HBE, I would tell you the end result you should be achieving by discussing goals, probably in numerical terms. But I couldn't tell you how you should achieve that result. I couldn't tell you what you as an individual must do to reach that level of management skill.

I am not in a position to make that kind of recommendation about weight management either. You are the only person who can decide if you need or want this kind of training.

You will continue to learn about yourself through using the system. Apparently you've already learned you do need some method of stress reduction, independent of food. This is fine. As long as you keep using the system, you will not fall back into the stress-eating syndrome for any long period of time. Whatever else you do to cope under stress is up to you.

Q. I am confused about one aspect of the stress connection. If emotional stress interferes with digestion and causes heartburn, why does it make us fat? Why doesn't the undigested food simply pass through?

A. A defective product still reaches the end of the assembly line, doesn't it?

Stress interferes with digestion, but does not prohibit it from taking place. Stress can make digestion of fats more difficult and can cause heartburn. This does not allow you to take in more fat while absorbing less calories. In fact, stress may have the reverse effect.

Your body may absorb *more* calories from the fats, in spite of its digestive problems, because stress also interferes with calorie burning. Stress increases fatty acid metabolism, blood glucose levels, and growth hormone production. So you get heartburn—but you also get fat.

Q. Is there a food I could eat to reduce stress?

A. Is there a quick-fix management solution for stress in the workplace? No. But sound management practices work together to reduce workplace stress and enable workers to cope more easily.

Many medical experts believe that a combination of weight control, sensible nutrition, and exercise does reduce stress. Three well-balanced meals, moderation and variety in food, low amounts of junk food, regular exercise—all are part of a sound management program.

Q. I think I eat out of boredom more than out of stress. Could this be true or am I once again kidding myself?

A. It could be true.

Some studies indicate workers make more mistakes when bored than when under stress. And medical authorities tell me that a common cause of overeating is using food as the means of avoiding unpleasant tasks or breaking from tedious routine. If you are eating out of boredom, you need to find ways to make your work and your life more interesting, more challenging. Again, you are learning a lot about yourself through using the Strategic Weight-Control System. As you continue working with it, you will gain even greater understanding.

Q. Everyone in my family is overweight to some extent. Until I learned about psychological roadblocks, I thought our family fatness was genetic. Now I wonder if it isn't psychological. What do you think?

A. I don't believe management is ever "genetic." Anyone can learn to manage.

Most medical experts now agree that a "tendency to fat" is not a genetic trait. In other words, we are not born to be fat. Fat "runs in families" because fat parents tend to overfeed babies and young children. Being fat is rewarded in those families. Overeating is a learned behavior.

If you were a fat baby, you were fat because your parents gave you too much food, not because you were born programmed to be fat. Overfeeding created more fat cells in your body than you need. But we've learned we can break free of the tyranny of those fat cells.

Breaking free of the tyranny of your family's behavior pattern may be more difficult, but you can do it. The system makes it possible for anyone to be an Effective Weight Manager, no matter what his or her past history, no matter how fat the family tree.

You are on your way to changing your life pattern now that you recognize it.

Q. I've been using the system for more than two months; and it's working. The added benefit, one I did not expect, is a tremendous increase in self-esteem. When I was fat, I had low self-esteem, though I wasn't aware of it. Do fat people feel so bad about themselves because our society makes us feel bad?

A. Bad managers feel unhappy in part because their peers, superiors, and subordinates know how inept they are. And certainly social pressure is a cause of the fat person's unhappiness with him or herself. Thin is valued in America, especially in the 1980s, a decade when so much emphasis has been placed on good health. It is not possible to be healthy and fat. So the fat person feels undesirable and unhealthy.

But some of that low esteem is self-generated too. We don't feel good about ourselves when we aren't in control of our lives. The bad manager doesn't need a memo signed by the entire staff to tell him he's doing a poor job. He knows it.

As long as we are unable to manage our weight, we are unable to *manage.* We feel inadequate at least to some degree. Managing well is really its own best reward, isn't it?

I am pleased when people congratulate me on my weight loss—and when my wife puts her arm around my waist and tells me she's glad the spare tire is gone. But the best part about managing my weight is the new way I feel about myself. Other people, and outside pressures, do affect us. The root of self-esteem, however, lies in oneself.

Q. Since I began using the Strategic Weight-Control System, I learned some surprising things about myself, mainly that I am seldom really hungry. Now that I only eat when I am hungry, I have no problem at all controlling my weight. Why do we kid ourselves so much about hunger?

A. Have you ever worked in a company where there were too many managers for the workload? They made busy work to justify their jobs and kidded themselves about their importance, didn't they?

Weight managers who have no system of accountability behave in the same fashion.

Unless we have such a system, it's very easy to kid ourselves about every aspect of weight management. We ignore our body's true hunger signals and refuse to eat appropriately. What we confuse with appetite for food is often a hunger for something that will alleviate stress, make us feel warm, protected, loved. When we stop using food as a buffer, a soother, a reward, and begin listening to the body's true hunger signals, we do eat natural amounts.

Q. Why don't doctors treat fat people? Either they ignore us or put us on diet and water pills.

A. No one, not even a doctor, can manage your weight for you. It's *your* job.

I suspect doctors don't "treat" fat people because they don't know how and because the success rate for weight loss is so low. If 95 percent of dieters regain the weight they lose, the doctors may feel the percentage of success doesn't justify their time and involvement in a patient's fat problem.

Many of the Control Group Team members have also told me their doctors said, "Lose weight," but were unable to tell them how to do it. They complained doctors were indifferent to the psychological problems of the over-weight. Most doctors send the patient home with a diet menu and tell him to come back in three months.

When it comes to treating obesity, most doctors are high-priced consultants without the ability to apply their knowledge to the job at hand.

Q. My husband has been doing everything he can to sabotage my weight-control program. He brings me candy and takes me to expensive restaurants. Why isn't he being helpful? Can I continue to lose if he doesn't want me to be thin?

A. If you were working with a close colleague on a company project, you would no doubt prefer to have that person's full support of your efforts—but lack of support wouldn't prevent you from fulfilling your obligation, would it? You would do your job, of course.

It's unfortunate that you aren't getting cooperation from your husband. He has his own hidden agenda in regard to your weight. It may be helpful for you to try to understand his agenda or it may not be. Most important, you must understand your own hidden agenda, your psychological roadblocks to being thin.

You *can* be an Effective Weight Manager with or without his "help." This is a system for the individual. You do not need support from anyone else. He is forcing you to make more food choices than you might like to make at this point, but he cannot force you to make choices you don't want to make. You are managing your weight; he is not.

Q. I have read that you should only eat when hungry

and not stick to a rigid meal schedule—but I have to start work at a certain hour, which regiments my breakfast time, and I have to take lunch at a certain hour too. It's really not possible in my circumstances to eat only when I'm hungry, is it?

A. *All* managers must manage within the confines of their jobs, their company's objectives, their departmental budgets. Very few people have absolute freedom to schedule their meals. Most of us are hemmed in by office hours, aren't we?

You may have a narrow time span in which to eat breakfast or lunch, but if you are not hungry during this time you do have some options. Can't you eat very lightly, perhaps saving part of breakfast or lunch for a coffee break snack? There are always ways to work within the routine if you want to find them. Don't use this as an excuse for not managing.

Q. You keep advising us to walk, especially when we're traveling. Will walking from hotel to restaurant really make that much difference?

A. Pretend you can invest money in three different plans, each one equally safe and accessible. The first gives you 5 percent return on your money, the next 6 percent, the last 7 percent. Which will you choose?

I choose to walk because walking gives me a greater return than not walking.

A man burns sixty calories per hour when asleep. A man on a diet burns fifty calories per hour asleep. But a man who exercises regularly burns seventy calories an hour asleep. Yes, walking—if you walk often and briskly—does make a difference.

Q. Traveling is still difficult for me in terms of weight management. I work very hard all day when I'm out of town. I usually begin with a breakfast meeting, have a business lunch, work through until a late dinner shared with associates. When I get back to my room at nine or ten, I am so tired and so full I can't move, let alone walk. I watch TV until I fall asleep. How do I get out of this trap?

A. I have known managers who will put in twelve-hour workdays and accomplish less than those who work eight or nine hours because they work less efficiently. You are still not working efficiently as a weight manager and exercising your options, are you?

You don't have to eat three heavy meals a day just because you're out of town on business. And you will have more energy if you take the time to walk from place to place. Exercise also invigorates the mind, which can make the time spent on business more productive. It's hard to do your best work when you feel lethargic and "stuffed" from eating too much, expending too little energy.

TV is the business person's enemy on the road. The worst management response you can make is to return to your hotel room after eating a large meal and sprawl in front of the TV set. Look at your options again. You are only trapped when you think you are.

Q. Airline food is the worst. How can you be an Effective Weight Manager and eat on an airplane?

A. You can be an Effective Weight Manager under any circumstances.

When you make flight reservations, order a special meal. Airlines serve vegetarian, seafood, low-cal, and other special plates. They are usually tastier than regular fare. But you can eat regular fare and still be an Effective Weight Manager.

Treat air travel as just another part of your life, one that presents more choices to be made—rather than as an excuse not to manage.

19

Communicating the System

"Preach not to others what they should eat, but
eat as becomes you, and be silent."
— Epictetus

A good idea is like a good investment.

When you have a good idea, other people want "in."
They want to hear the details and share the success. The
Strategic Weight-Control System has worked so well for
me and for other members of the Control Group Team
that we've found ourselves sharing it with family and
friends—at their request.

The system is designed for the individual. It is not
necessary, of course, that you share it with anyone. If
other members of your family do adopt the system, they
will be using it as individuals too. Each of you will be an
Effective Weight Manager in charge of your own weight-
management program. You won't be part of some family
version of Weight Watchers. Your success will never be
dependent on the success of anyone else. And if you
coerce your spouse to begin the program, he or she will
probably not make a real commitment to it and thus may
not succeed.

Still, many of you will probably hand this book to a

spouse, sibling, or friend simply because you have found a good idea and they have asked for the details. Some members of the Control Group Team have spouses who have been using the system as long, or almost as long, as they have. Others say their spouses didn't want "in" until they saw visible signs of success.

We have seen how family behavioral patterns can affect our attitudes toward weight control in a negative way. Well, introducing the system to family members can have a positive effect. If you can be the catalyst that inspires someone in your family to become an Effective Weight Manager, you may be changing those patterns for several family members, not just for yourself. You're probably very excited about the system and anxious to do just that.

Some of the Control Group Team members are particularly anxious to create new behavioral models for their children. They grew up in families where being fat was being normal. They want different standards for their own children.

"I want my kids to have the example of good eating habits," one woman told me. "I want them to grow up knowing good nutrition from bad, knowing how to use food in a healthy way, not in a sick way as a coping mechanism. And I want them to exercise."

Certainly that is a laudable ambition.

I have seen firsthand what good examples can accomplish in a family. Recently, when our daughter married, she wore my wife's wedding gown. That in itself isn't unusual: Some young women do wear their mother's gown. But, before turning the dress over to the bride, June tried it on; and it fit. I was proud of her for managing her weight so successfully that she could still wear her wedding gown today.

And my own success with the system has inspired a

daughter-in-law to become an Effective Weight Manager. She too is in charge of her weight now. I'm glad I was able to share the system with her, to give her the tool she needed to manage.

But we all have to be careful about *how* we involve our families in the system. We can't take responsibility for someone else's management program. We can only lend the book, introduce the idea, share our experiences.

In their enthusiasm, some of the Control Group Team members have tried to force the Effective Weight Manager program on spouses. One says, "I learned that you can't be anyone else's weight-control keeper. My wife stayed on the program for a very short time because she had never made the decision to manage for herself. She followed me all the way. I made her weigh herself in the mornings; I recorded the weights for her. I kept her notebook and chart.

"Well, after a few weeks, I realized I was doing her program. She wasn't. It couldn't work that way; and it wasn't. I hope someday she decides for her own sake to manage her weight, but I know now I can't make her manage."

Another woman says she regards "spreading the word about the system a form of networking. When you network, you let people know about opportunities that exist. You don't force them to take advantage of the opportunities. You only share information. I am willing to share the system with anyone, but I don't push it."

We have all learned that being an Effective Weight Manager is an individual responsibility. Like all good managers, we have built-in leadership capabilities. An important leadership function is to set the right example. For Effective Weight Managers, example setting may be the *only* leadership function.

If you can be an Effective Weight Manager and set a

good example for your family, good for you. But please regard that example as the by-product, not the main product, of managing. It is an added benefit, not a goal, of your personal management plan.

When other family members do decide to use the system, don't get involved in their personal goal setting. Don't give them a voice in yours. You can't chastise them for choices made that you believe are wrong—or praise them when you think they've made the "right" choices. Admire the results, not the process. Each person is autonomous. A family cannot share the system the way they might share a thirty-day diet plan.

Some Control Group Team members say their spouses who use the system have become exercise partners too, which is another nice by-product of the management process.

"I couldn't convince my husband to take walks with me until he started using the system," one woman told me. "Now he is very conscious of energy expenditure; and he likes walking."

And when both spouses are Effective Weight Managers, one doesn't have to worry about the other's sabotage efforts. Two weight managers might adopt certain habits, like filling plates in the kitchen rather than from bowls at the table, or they may agree not to purchase snack foods at the grocery. This commingling of managerial functions can "help" at home by creating a controlled environment where goals are more easily pursued.

But there is a downside to all this cooperation, just as there would be a downside to mutual dependence in the workplace.

An Effective Weight Manager who becomes too accustomed to help in making choices at home may find it harder to make choices outside the home alone. That's why I keep reminding people—when I know both spouses are using the system—that this is an *individual* program. Each Effective Weight Manager is responsible for his or her own weight. You are always managing independently. And this is true, no matter how many independent Effective Weight Managers are living together under your roof.

When a family member asks about the system, share it. But treat the family member exactly as you would treat a new colleague at the office. You would offer to show him around and answer questions for a reasonable period of time, but you wouldn't offer to do his work, to take on his responsibilities in addition to your own.

Likewise, the family member is a peer who is taking on a job comparable to yours. He or she deserves your respect in the same way a new colleague in the workplace does. If you do get too closely involved in the other person's job, both of you are going to be in trouble.

Some people tell me the sense of "competition" between them and their spouse helped them lose weight. But I remind them management is not a competitive sport. If two managers are competing in the workplace, they will eventually be neglecting work they should be doing because they are concentrating on high-visibility tasks, those tasks that can be measured and compared.

Emphasis should not be placed on who can lose the most pounds. Using the system this way distorts its purpose. Just as each of us sets professional goals for the good of the organization and for our own personal growth, we set weight-management goals for the overall health of the body and our personal sense of how we want to look. We don't set our goals in relation to anyone else's goals.

I believe strongly in the individual, in what each of us can accomplish alone once we take charge of our lives. As an Effective Weight Manager, you too have become a rugged individualist. The best advice you can give family or friends who want to use the system is to convey this message.

Don't help them. Don't take responsibility for their weight control. And remember, just as you don't need them for success, they don't need you either.

They can, and will, manage successfully on their own.

20

Sustaining Dynamic Performance

"Success is a journey, not a destination."
—Ben Sweetland

Once I had achieved my weight-loss goals, I felt the same way I do whenever a large project has been brought to completion: proud, satisfied, *successful*. When a new Adam's Mark Hotel is finished, for example, I feel for a brief period of time as if everything that needed to be done has been done. And that is a good feeling. It lasts, oh, perhaps for several hours. Then I begin to focus on other projects, get excited about new ideas, new goals.

As an Effective Weight Manager, my goal for life is weight maintenance. When you compare maintenance to weight loss, maintenance does not appear to be a dramatic or interesting process. Building a hotel looks more exciting than maintaining one, doesn't it? During construction, the progress is evident. But after that hotel is open for the business of accommodating guests, "progress" is all behind the scenes. We expect the rooms, service, food, to be high-quality. We would only notice if they weren't. The work that goes into maintaining progress isn't visible to us most of the time.

So it is with weight maintenance—a straight line on

the chart, a set of numbers that should not vary greatly from day to day, week to week. As long as the lines and numbers reflect a constant level of high performance, they are no longer noteworthy.

Will the numbers be enough to sustain my interest—and yours—for the rest of our lives?

I believe they will. The test of management is performance, the achievement of goals. A good manager never reaches a point where there is nothing more to achieve, no more goals to set. The numbers may not excite anyone else, but they excite him because he knows exactly what they mean—sustained performance.

Maintenance appears less dramatic, yet it is the far greater challenge. We know the odds against maintaining loss: 95 percent of those who lose regain within two years. Compared to maintaining, losing is easy.

And the Effective Weight Manager who is managing maintenance doesn't have the same incentives he had as a manager in charge of loss.

When I first began losing weight, I was encouraged by the line sloping down the chart, the numbers in my notebook growing smaller, the compliments from co-workers, friends, and family. Now that line remains stable, the numbers fluctuate very little. And people who know me have adjusted to my new size. They no longer say, "Fred, you've lost weight; you're looking good!"

Perhaps this absence of incentives, in part, is what leads many who have lost to regain. If I did not have the Strategic Weight-Control System, the same thing might happen to me when people stopped praising my weight loss. But I do have the system; and so do you. As Effective Weight Managers, we are not dependent on external incentives. We do not react to circumstances. We *manage*.

I have come to regard the Strategic Weight-Control System as the mechanism of management, the tool that will keep me on track. Just as a business organization cannot function without a management structure, a weight-management program cannot either. As long as I continue to set new goals *and* to rely on the mechanism, I cannot fail. Nor can you.

The Control Group Team members also recognize the importance of continuing to use the system after their weight-loss goals have been met.

Some of them have decided to break their maintenance goals into quarterly period goals. They have said to themselves, "I have lost the weight I wanted to lose so my long-term goal is continuous maintenance. But for now I will concentrate on the short term: maintaining this weight, this straight line across the chart, for the next three months."

They believe the long-term goal is more manageable when viewed this way. And they have prepared charts in three-month segments to help them manage.

Others have learned so much about themselves through a careful reading of the numbers in their notebooks that they have decided to express maintenance goals in terms of those notebook numbers.

One woman says her weight will fluctuate by as much as four pounds during the month due to water retention. Her goal, then, is to keep her weight within the confines of a four-pound spread.

However you decide to express your maintenance goals is up to you. The system guarantees that you will be able to meet them, that you will be able to sustain the dynamic performance you have begun as an Effective Weight Manager.

If you are anything like me, you need constant new challenges. You quickly get bored with repeating tasks, even if the tasks are rewarding. Maintenance is *not* a series of repetitive tasks. We will be continuously striving to match our own performance records; and we will be constantly confronted with new choices.

I cannot predict the challenges I will face in weight management. Nor can you. As I continue to age, my body may require less food to sustain its weight; and so I may have to make adjustments to my weight-control equation, eating different kinds and amounts of food, increasing energy expenditure. Or there may be a time when a physical illness or infirmity limits my energy expenditure for a time. Maybe I'll sprain an ankle skiing and have to forego walking for weeks. I know that whatever happens in the future I will be able to maintain my weight through using the system, adjusting the equation to fit the circumstances of the moment. I will manage the external forces. They will never manage me.

Will you be one of those who manage—or will you be managed?

□ APPENDIX I □

Building the Control Group Team

T he Control Group Team members were *The Effective Weight Manager's* test pilots. This group was vital to the writing of the book because we needed to prove that many other people could use the Strategic Weight-Control System and lose weight or maintain a loss. They provided necessary background information for the book by sharing their weight-management problems and experiences.

The majority of the team members were HBE employees, though a large number were from the outside: friends, relatives, business associates. Our "team" was actually far-flung, including a New York City editor who lost the ten pounds he's been talking about losing for ten years and a Los Angeles attorney who lost thirty pounds. And some of the team began using the system to maintain a loss, including one man who maintained his weight at the same level for three months, the first time he had ever been able to keep the weight off for longer than a few weeks.

With the help of my corporate communications department, I collected information about the group through an informal and loosely structured network. We proceeded as follows:

1. A general companywide memo was sent to all employees informing them that material explaining a weight-loss system would be available to anyone who wanted it.

2. We held a short meeting after work in the company cafeteria to explain the purpose of the control group and distribute packets of material, which later became chapters of this book. Each packet included a questionnaire.

3. Those who wished to be interviewed filled out and returned the questionnaire to the communications department. (We had far more responses than we had anticipated.)

4. Periodically we called them or they contacted one of us to report progress or ask questions. Some informal lunch meetings were also held. These meetings were not support or therapy sessions. They were held primarily as a convenient means of gathering information for the book.

We never attempted to make the Control Group Team a support group. No one was coerced to continue using the system. Commitment to the program was individual and voluntary.

Not all those who returned questionnaires decided to use the system. Some used it for brief periods, a few days to two weeks, reported no weight loss, and discontinued using it. Everyone who stayed with the system for at least six weeks did lose weight.

If you distribute copies of *The Effective Weight Manager* to your employees as a special benefit of your health care plan, please do so in the same spirit. This is a plan for the individual. Success in weight management, as in business, depends solely on the manager.

·APPENDIX II·

Strategic Weight-Control Graph

Fred Kummer's Graph

	Nov. 26 to Dec. 2 Week 1	Dec. 3 to Dec. 9 Week 2	Dec. 10 to Dec. 16 Week 3	Dec. 17 to Dec. 23 Week 4	Dec. 24 to Dec. 30 Week 5	Dec. 31 to Jan. 6 Week 6
M	188.00	184.00	181.50	181.00	178.75	178.00
T	186.50	183.50	182.00	181.00	178.50	178.00
W	185.50	183.00	181.75	180.75	179.00	179.00
T	185.00	—	181.00	180.00	—	179.00
F	185.00	184.00	180.25	179.00	178.50	177.75
S	185.50	183.00	181.00	178.50	180.00	176.75
S	184.75	183.00	180.25	178.00	178.00	176.75
	1300.25	1100.50	1267.75	1258.25	1072.75	1245.25
Average Wt.	185.75	183.42	181.11	179.75	178.79	177.89
Loss	0	2.33	2.31	1.36	.96	.90
Total Loss	0	2.33	4.64	6.00	6.96	7.86
Avg. Loss Wk.	—	2.33	2.32	2.00	1.74	1.57

Jan. 7 to Jan. 13 Week 7	Jan. 14 to Jan. 20 Week 8	Jan. 21 to Jan. 27 Week 9	Jan. 28 to Feb. 3 Week 10	Feb. 4 to Feb. 10 Week 11	Feb. 11 to Feb. 17 Week 12
—	177.25	—	175.50	174	173.25
177.75	—	—	176.00	174	173
177.00	—	176.25	175.75	174.50	—
—	177.00	174.00	174.00	174	173.50
176.00	177.00	175.25	173.00	173	172.50
176.25	175.00	174.50	174.25	172.50	172
176.50	173.00	175.75	174.25	172.50	172
883.50	879.25	875.75	1222.75	1214.25	1035.25
176.70	175.85	175.15	174.68	173.46	172.54
1.19	.85	.70	.47	1.22	.92
9.05	9.90	10.60	11.07	12.29	13.21
1.51	1.41	1.33	1.23	1.22	1.20

	Week 1		Week 2		Week 3		Week 4		Week 5		Week 6	
Current Weight												
5 lbs.												
10 lbs.												
15 lbs.												
20 lbs.												
25 lbs.												
M												
T												
W												
T												
F												
S												
S												
Average Wt.												
Loss												
Total Loss												
Avg. Loss Wk.												

Week 7		Week 8		Week 9		Week 10		Week 11		Week 12